A FEAST OF INFORMATION—
for people who love to eat but need to know
the calorie count of their meals.

BARBARA KRAUS 1990 CALORIE GUIDE
TO BRAND NAMES AND BASIC FOODS
lists thousands of basic and ready-to-eat foods,
from appetizers to desserts—carry it to the
supermarket, to the restaurant, to the beach, to
the coffee cart, and on trips.

Flip through these fact-filled pages. Mix, match,
and keep track of calories as they add up. But
remember, strawberry shortcake is fattening any
way you slice it!

BARBARA KRAUS
1990 Calorie
Guide to
Brand Names and
Basic Foods

Barbara Kraus
1990 Calorie
Guide to
Brand Names and
Basic Foods

A SIGNET BOOK

NEW AMERICAN LIBRARY

A DIVISION OF PENGUIN BOOKS USA INC.

For Michael & James Molina

Copyright © 1971, 1973, 1975, 1976, 1977 by Barbara Kraus
© 1978 by John R. Fernbach, Esq. and Murray Cohen,
Co-Executors to the Estate of Barbara Kraus.
Copyright © 1979, 1980, 1981, 1982, 1983, 1984, 1985, 1986, 1987, 1988, 1989
by New American Library a division of Penguin Books USA INC.

Excerpted from *Dictionary of Calories and Carbohydrates*

SIGNET, SIGNET CLASSIC, MENTOR, ONYX, PLUME,
MERIDIAN AND NAL BOOKS
are published by New American Library, a division of Penguin Books
USA Inc., 1633 Broadway, New York, New York 10019

FIRST PRINTING, JANUARY, 1990

1 2 3 4 5 6 7 8 9

PRINTED IN THE UNITED STATES OF AMERICA

Foreword

The composition of the foods we eat is not static: it changes from time to time. In the case of *brand-name* products, manufacturers alter their recipes to reflect the availability of ingredients, advances in technology, or improvements in formulae. Each year new products appear on the market and some old ones are discontinued.

On the other hand, information on *basic foods* such as meats, vegetables, and fruits may also change as a result of the development of better analytical methods, different growing conditions, or new marketing practices. These changes, however, are usually relatively small as compared with those in manufactured products.

Some differences may be found between the values in this book and those appearing on the product labels. This is usually due to the fact that the Food and Drug Administration permits manufacturers to round the figures reported on labels. The data in this book are reported as calculated without rounding. If large differences between the two sets of values are noted, they may be due to changes in product formulae, and in those cases the label data should be used.

For all these reasons, a book of calorie or nutritive values of foods must be kept up to date by a periodic reviewing and revision of the data presented.

Therefore, this handy calorie counter will provide each year the most current and accurate estimates available. Generous use of this little book will help you and your family to select the right foods and the proper number of calories each member requires to gain, lose, or maintain healthy and attractive weight.

Barbara Kraus

Why This Book?

Some of the data presented here can be found in more detail in my bestselling *Calories and Carbohydrates,* a dictionary of 8,000 brand names and basic foods. Complete as it is, it is meant to be used as a reference book at home or in the office and not to be squeezed into a suit jacket or evening bag—it's just too big.

Therefore, responding to the need for a portable calorie guide, and one which can reflect food changes often, I have written this smaller and handier version. The selection of material and the additional new entries provide readers with pertinent data on thousands of products that they would prepare at home to take to work, eat in a restaurant or luncheonette, nibble on from the coffee cart, take to the beach, buy in the candy store, et cetera.

For the sake of saving space and providing you with a greater selection of products, I had to make certain compromises: whereas in the giant book there are several physical descriptions of a product, here there is but one.

For Beginners Only

The language of dieting is no more difficult to learn than any other new subject; in many respects, it's much easier, particularly if you restrict your education to clearly defined goals.

For you who never before had the need or the interest in a lesson in weight control, I offer the following elementary introduction, applicable to any diet, self-initiated or suggested by your doctor, nutritionist, or dietician.

A Calorie

An analysis of foods in terms of calories is most often the chosen method to describe the relative energy yielded by foods.

A calorie is a shorthand way to summarize the units of energy contained in any foodstuff or alcoholic beverage, similar to the way a thermometer indicates heat. One pound of fat is equal to 3,500 calories. Add this number of calories to those you need to balance your energy requirements and you will gain one pound; subtract it and you will lose a pound.

Other Nutrients

Carbohydrates—which include sugars, starches, and acids—are only one of several chemical compounds in foods that yield calories. Proteins, found mainly in beef, poultry, and fish; fats, found in oils, butter, marbling of meat, and poultry skin; and alcohol, found in some beverages, also contribute calories. Except for alcohol, most foods contain at least some of these nutrients.

The amount of carbohydrates varies from zero in meats and a trace in alcohol to a heavy concentration in sugar, syrups, some fruits, grains, and root vegetables.

As of this date, the most respected nutritional researchers insist that some carbohydrate is necessary every day for maintaining good health. The amount to be included is an individual matter, and in any drastic effort to change your eating patterns, be sure to consult your doctor first.

Now, on how to use this new language.

To begin with, you use this book like a dictionary. If your plan is to cut down on calories, the easiest way to do so is to consult the portable calorie counter and keep an accurate count of your total intake of food and beverages for a period of seven days. If you have not gained or lost weight during that week, divide that number by seven and you'll have your maintenance diet expressed in calories. To lose weight, you must reduce your daily or weekly intake of calories below this maintenance level. (To gain, increase the intake.)

Keeping in mind that you want to stay healthy and eat well-balanced meals (which include the basic food groups: milk or milk products; meat, poultry, or fish; vegetables and fruits; and whole grain or enriched breads or cereals, as well as some fats or oils), you then start to cut down on your portion in order to reduce your intake of calories. There are many imaginative ways to diet without total withdrawal from one's favorite foods.

Once you know and don't have to guess what calories are in your foods, you can relax and enjoy them. It could turn out that dieting isn't so bad after all.

ABBREVIATIONS AND SYMBOLS

* = prepared as package directs[1]
< = less than
& = and
" = inch
canned = bottles or jars as well as cans
dia. = diameter
fl. = fluid
liq. = liquid
lb. = pound
med. = medium

oz. = ounce
pkg. = package
pt. = pint
qt. = quart
sq. = square
T. = tablespoon
Tr. = trace
tsp. = teaspoon
wt. = weight

Italics or name in parentheses = registered trademark, ®. All data not identified by company or trademark are based on material obtained from the United States Department of Agriculture or Health, Education and Welfare/Food and Agriculture Organization.

EQUIVALENTS

By Weight
1 pound = 16 ounces
1 ounce = 28.35 grams
3.52 ounces = 100 grams

By Volume
1 quart = 4 cups
1 cup = 8 fluid ounces
1 cup = ½ pint
1 cup = 16 tablespoons
2 tablespoons = 1 fluid ounce
1 tablespoon = 3 teaspoons
1 pound butter = 4 sticks or 2 cups

[1]If the package directions call for whole or skim milk, the data given here are for whole milk unless otherwise stated.

A

Food and Description	Measure or Quantity	Calories
ABALONE, canned	4 oz.	91
AC'CENT	¼ tsp.	3
AGNOLETTI, frozen (Buitoni):		
Cheese filled	2-oz. serving	196
Meat filled	2-oz. serving	206
ALBACORE, raw, meat only	4 oz.	201
ALLSPICE (French's)	1 tsp.	6
ALMOND:		
In shell	10 nuts	60
Shelled, raw, natural, with skins	1 oz.	170
Roasted, dry (Planters)	1 oz.	170
Roasted, oil (Tom's)	1 oz.	180
ALMOND EXTRACT (Durkee) pure	1 tsp.	13
ALPHA-BITS, cereal (Post)	1 cup (1 oz.)	110
AMARETTO DI SARONNO	1 fl. oz.	83
ANCHOVY, PICKLED, canned, flat or rolled, not heavily salted, drained (Granadaisa)	2-oz. can	80
ANISE EXTRACT (Durkee) imitation	1 tsp.	16
ANISETTE:		
(DeKuyper)	1 fl. oz.	95
(Mr. Boston)	1 fl. oz.	88
APPLE:		
Fresh, with skin	2½" dia.	61
Fresh, without skin	2½" dia.	53
Canned:		
(Comstock):		
Rings, drained	1 ring	30
Sliced	⅙ of 21-oz. can	45
(White House):		
Rings	1 ring	25
Sliced	½ cup (4 oz.)	54
Dried:		
(Del Monte)	1 cup	140
(Sun-Maid/Sunsweet)	2-oz. serving	150
Frozen, sweetened	1 cup	325
APPLE BROWN BETTY	1 cup	325
APPLE BUTTER:		
(Home Brands)	1 T.	52

1

Food and Description	Measure or Quantity	Calories
(Smucker's)	1 T.	38
(White House)	1 oz.	50
APPLE CHERRY BERRY DRINK,		
canned (Lincoln)	6 fl. oz.	90
APPLE CIDER:		
Canned:		
(Johanna Farms)	½ cup	56
(Mott's) sweet	½ cup	59
(Tree Top)	6 fl. oz.	90
*Mix, *Country Time*	8 fl. oz.	98
APPLE-CRANBERRY DRINK		
(Hi-C):		
Canned	6 fl. oz.	90
*Mix	6 fl. oz.	72
APPLE-CRANBERRY JUICE,		
canned (Lincoln)	6 fl. oz.	100
APPLE DRINK:		
Canned:		
Capri Sun, natural	6¾ fl. oz.	90
(Hi-C)	6 fl. oz.	92
Ssips (Johanna Farms)	8.45-fl.-oz. container	130
*Mix (Hi-C)	6 fl. oz.	72
APPLE DUMPLINGS, frozen		
(Pepperidge Farm)	1 dumpling	260
APPLE, ESCALLOPED:		
Canned (White House)	½ cup (4.5 oz.)	156
Frozen (Stouffer's)	4 oz.	140
APPLE-GRAPE JUICE, canned:		
(Musselman's)	6 fl. oz.	82
(Red Cheek)	6 fl. oz.	69
APPLE JACKS, cereal (Kellogg's)	1 cup (1 oz.)	110
APPLE JAM (Smucker's)	1 T.	53
APPLE JELLY:		
Sweetened:		
(Bama)	1 T.	45
(Home Brands)	1 T.	52
(Smucker's)	1 T.	67
Dietetic:		
(Estee; Featherweight;		
Louis Sherry)	1 T.	6
(Diet Delight)	1 T.	12
APPLE JUICE:		
Canned:		
(Borden) *Sippin' Pak*	8.45-fl.-oz. container	110
(Johanna Farms) *Tree Ripe*	8.45-fl.-oz. container	121
(Lincoln)	6 fl. oz.	90
(Red Cheek)	6 fl. oz.	85
(Thank You Brand)	6 fl. oz.	82

Food and Description	Measure or Quantity	Calories
(Tree Top) regular	6 fl. oz.	90
(White House)	6 fl. oz.	87
Chilled (Minute Maid)	6 fl. oz.	100
*Frozen:		
(Minute Maid)	6 fl. oz.	100
(Seneca Foods) Vitamin C added	6 fl. oz.	90
(Tree Top)	6 fl. oz.	90
APPLE JUICE DRINK, canned		
(Sunkist)	8.5 fl. oz.	140
APPLE PIE (See PIE, Apple)		
APPLE RAISIN CRISP, cereal		
(Kellogg's)	⅔ cup	130
APPLE SAUCE:		
Regular:		
(Del Monte)	½ cup	90
(Hunt's) *Snack Pak:*		
Regular	4¼ oz.	50
Raspberry	4¼ oz.	80
(Mott's):		
Regular, jarred:		
Regular	6 oz.	150
Cinnamon	6 oz.	152
Single-serve cups:		
Regular	4 oz.	100
Cherry	3¾ oz.	72
Peach	3¾ oz.	75
Strawberry	3¾ oz.	76
(Thank You Brand)	½ cup	87
(Tree Top) Natural	½ cup	60
(White House) regular or chunky	½ cup	100
Dietetic:		
(Del Monte, Lite; Diet Delight)	½ cup	50
(Mott's) Single-serve cups	4 oz.	53
(S&W) *Nutradiet*, white		
or blue label	½ cup	55
(Thank You Brand)	½ cup	54
(White House)	½ cup	59
APPLE STRUDEL, frozen		
(Pepperidge Farm)	3 oz.	240
APRICOT:		
Fresh, whole	1 apricot	18
Canned, regular pack:		
(Del Monte) whole, or halves,		
peeled	½ cup	200
(Stokely-Van Camp)	1 cup	220
Canned, dietetic, solids & liq.:		
(Del Monte) Lite	½ cup	64
(Diet Delight):		
Juice pack	½ cup	60

3

Water pack	½ cup	35
(Featherweight):		
Juice pack	½ cup	50
Water pack	½ cup	35
(Libby's) Lite	½ cup	60
(S&W) *Nutradiet:*		
Halves, white or blue label	½ cup	50
Whole, juice	½ cup	40
Dried:		
(Del Monte; Sun-Maid; Sunsweet)	2 oz.	140
APRICOT & PINEAPPLE		
PRESERVE OR JAM:		
Sweetened:		
(Home Brands)	1 T.	52
(Smucker's)	1 T.	53
Dietetic:		
(Diet Delight; Louis Sherry)	1 T.	6
(S&W) *Nutradiet*	1 T.	12
APRICOT LIQUEUR (DeKuyper)	1 fl. oz.	82
APRICOT NECTAR:		
(Del Monte)	6 fl. oz.	100
(Libby's)	6 fl. oz.	110
APRICOT-PINEAPPLE NECTAR,		
canned, dietetic (S&W) *Nutradiet,*		
blue label	6 oz.	35
APRICOT PRESERVE:		
Sweetened (Home Brands)	1 T.	51
Dietetic (Estee)	1 T.	6
ARBY'S:		
Bac'n Cheddar Deluxe	1 sandwich	561
Beef & Cheddar Sandwich	1 sandwich	490
Chicken breast sandwich	7¼-oz. sandwich	592
Croissant:		
Bacon & egg	1 croissant	420
Butter	1 croissant	220
Chicken salad	1 croissant	460
Ham & Swiss	1 croissant	330
Mushroom & Swiss	1 croissant	340
Sausage & egg	1 croissant	530
French fries	1½-oz. serving	211
Ham 'N Cheese	1 sandwich	353
Potato cakes	2 pieces	201
Potato, stuffed:		
Broccoli & cheddar	1 potato	541
Deluxe	1 potato	648
Mushroom & cheese	1 potato	506
Taco	1 potato	619
Roast Beef:		
Regular	5 oz.	353

Food and Description	Measure or Quantity	Calories
Junior	3 oz.	218
King	6.7 oz.	467
Super	9¼ oz.	501
Garden salad (no dressing)	1 serving	165
Chef's salad (no dressing)	1 serving	235
Cashew chicken salad (contains dressing)	1 serving	505
Crackers	1 packet	25
Croutons	1 packet	70
Dressings:		
Blue cheese	1 packet	390
Buttermilk	1 packet	460
Honey French	1 packet	350
Light Italian	1 packet	25
ARTICHOKE:		
Boiled	15-oz. artichoke	187
Canned (Cara Mia) marinated, drained	6-oz. jar	175
Frozen (Birds Eye) deluxe	3 oz.	30
ASPARAGUS:		
Boiled	1 spear (½" dia. at base)	3
Canned, regular pack, solid & liq.:		
(Del Monte) spears, green or white	½ cup	20
(Green Giant)	8-oz. can	46
Canned, dietetic, solids & liq.:		
(Diet Delight)	½ cup	16
(Featherweight) cut spears	1 cup	40
(S&W) *Nutradiet*	1 cup	40
Frozen:		
(Birds Eye):		
Cuts	⅓ pkg.	25
Spears, regular or jumbo deluxe	⅓ pkg.	25
(Frosty Acres)	3.3 oz.	25
(Green Giant) cuts, butter sauce	3 oz.	57
(McKenzie)	⅓ pkg.	25
(Stouffer's) souffle	⅓ pkg.	115
ASPARAGUS PUREE, canned (Larsen)	½ cup	22
AUNT JEMIMA SYRUP (See SYRUP)		
AVOCADO, all varieties	1 fruit (10.7 oz.)	378
AWAKE (Birds Eye)	6 fl. oz.	84
AYDS:		
Butterscotch	1 piece	27
Chocolate, chocolate mint, vanilla	1 piece	26

B

Food and Description	Measure or Quantity	Calories
BACON, broiled:		
(Hormel) *Black Label*	1 slice	30
(Oscar Mayer):		
Regular slice	6-gram slice	35
Center cut	1 slice	24
Thick slice	1 slice	64
BACON BITS:		
Bac*Os (Betty Crocker)	1 tsp.	13
(French's) imitation	1 tsp.	6
(Hormel)	1 tsp.	10
(Libby's) crumbles	1 tsp.	8
(Oscar Mayer) real	1 tsp.	7
BACON, CANADIAN, unheated:		
(Eckrich)	1 oz.	35
(Hormel):		
Regular	1 slice	45
Light & Lean	1 slice	17
(Oscar Mayer) 93% fat free:		
Thin	.7-oz. slice	30
Thick	1-oz. slice	35
BACON, SIMULATED, cooked:		
(Oscar Mayer) *Lean'N Tasty*:		
Beef	1 strip	46
Pork	1 strip	54
(Swift's) *Sizzlean*, pork	1 strip	35
BAGEL (Lender's):		
Plain:		
Regular	1 bagel	150
Bagelette	1 bagel	70
Egg	1 bagel	150
Onion	1 bagel	160
Poppy seed	1 bagel	160
Raisin & honey	1 bagel	200
BAKING POWDER:		
(Calumet)	1 tsp.	2
(Davis)	1 tsp.	7
(Featherweight) low sodium, cereal free	1 tsp.	8

Food and Description	Measure or Quantity	Calories
BAMBOO SHOOTS:		
Raw, trimmed	4 oz.	31
Canned, drained (Chun King)	½ cup	32
BANANA, medium (Dole)	6.3-oz. banana (weighed unpeeled)	101
BANANA EXTRACT (Durkee) imitation	1 tsp.	15
BANANA NECTAR (Libby's)	6 fl. oz.	60
BANANA PIE (See PIE, Banana)		
BARBECUE SEASONING (French's)	1 tsp.	6
BARBERA WINE (Louis M. Martini) 12½% alcohol	3 fl. oz.	65
BARLEY, pearled (Quaker Scotch)	¼ cup	172
BASIL (French's)	1 tsp.	3
BASS:		
Baked, stuffed	3½″ × 4½″ × 1½″	531
Oven-fried	8¾″ × 4½″ × ⅝″	392
BAY LEAF (French's)	1 tsp.	5
B & B LIQUEUR	1 fl. oz.	94
B.B.Q. SAUCE & BEEF, frozen (Banquet) *Cookin' Bag*, sliced	4-oz. serving	133
BEAN, BAKED:		
(USDA):		
With pork & molasses sauce	1 cup	382
With pork & tomato sauce	1 cup	311
Canned:		
(Allens) *Wagon Master*	1 cup	260
(B&M) *Brick Oven*:		
Pea bean with pork in brown sugar sauce	8 oz.	300
Red kidney bean in brown sugar sauce	8 oz.	290
Vegetarian	8 oz.	250
(Campbell):		
Home style	8-oz. can	270
With pork & tomato sauce	8-oz. can	240
(Friend's):		
Pea	9-oz. serving	360
Yellow eye	9-oz. serving	360
(Furman's) & pork, in tomato sauce	8 oz.	245
(Grandma Brown's)	8 oz.	289
(Hormel) *Short Orders*, with bacon	7½-oz. can	330
(Hunt's) & pork	8 oz.	280
BEAN, BARBECUE (Campbell)	7⅞-oz. can	678

Food and Description	Measure or Quantity	Calories
BEAN & BEEF BURRITO DINNER, frozen (Swanson)	15¼-oz. dinner	720
BEAN, BLACK OR BROWN:		
Dry	1 cup	678
Canned (Goya) black	1 cup.	250
BEAN, CHILI, canned (Hunt's)	½ cup	90
BEAN, FAVA, canned (Progresso)	4 oz.	90
BEAN & FRANKFURTER, canned:		
(Campbell) in tomato and molasses sauce	7⅞-oz. can	360
(Hormel) *Short Orders,* 'n wieners	7½-oz. can	280
BEAN & FRANKFURTER DINNER, frozen:		
(Banquet)	10¼-oz. dinner	500
(Swanson)	12½-oz. dinner	550
BEAN, GARBANZO, canned:		
Regular (*Old El Paso*)	½ cup	77
Dietetic (S&W) *Nutradiet,* low sodium, green label	½ cup	105
BEAN, GREEN:		
Boiled, 1½" to 2" pieces, drained	½ cup	17
Canned, regular pack, solids & liq.:		
(Allen's):		
Whole	½ cup	21
With dry shelled beans	½ cup	40
(Del Monte)	4 oz.	20
(Green Giant) French or whole	½ cup	21
(Larsen) *Freshlike*	½ cup	20
Canned, dietetic, solids & liq.:		
(Del Monte) No Salt Added	4 oz.	19
(Diet Delight; S&W, *Nutradiet*)	½ cup	20
(Larsen) *Fresh-Lite*	½ cup	20
Frozen:		
(Birds Eye):		
Cut or French	⅓ pkg.	25
French, with almonds	3 oz.	50
Whole, deluxe	3 oz.	25
(Frosty Acres)	3 oz.	30
(Green Giant):		
Cut or French, with butter sauce	½ cup	40
Cut, *Harvest Fresh*	½ cup	25
(Larsen)	3 oz.	25
(Seabrook Farms; Southland)	⅓ pkg.	29
BEAN, GREEN & MUSHROOM CASSEROLE (Stouffer's)	½ pkg.	150
BEAN, GREEN, WITH POTATOES, canned (Sunshine) solids & liq.	½ cup	34

Food and Description	Measure or Quantity	Calories
BEAN, ITALIAN:		
Canned (Del Monte) solids & liq.	4 oz.	25
Frozen:		
(Birds Eye)	3 oz.	30
(Frosty Acres; Larsen)	3 oz.	30
BEAN, KIDNEY:		
Canned, regular pack, solids & liq.:		
(Allen's) red	½ cup	110
(Furman) red, fancy, light	½ cup	121
(Goya):		
Red	½ cup	115
White	½ cup	100
(Hunt's):		
Regular	½ cup (3.5 oz.)	80
Small	4 oz.	120
(Progresso)	½ cup	95
(Van Camp):		
Light	8 oz.	194
New Orleans style	8 oz.	188
Red	8 oz.	213
Canned, dietetic (S&W) *Nutradiet*, low sodium,	½ cup	90
BEAN, LIMA:		
Boiled, drained	½ cup	94
Canned, regular pack, solids & liq.:		
(Allen's):		
Regular	½ cup	60
Baby butter	½ cup	55
(Del Monte)	4 oz.	70
(Furman's)	½ cup	92
(Larsen) *Freshlike*	½ cup	80
(Sultana) butter bean	¼ of 15-oz. can	82
Canned, dietetic (Featherweight)	½ cup	80
Frozen:		
(Birds Eye) baby	⅓ pkg.	130
(Frosty Acres):		
Baby	3.3 oz.	130
Butter	3.2 oz.	140
Fordhook	3.3 oz.	100
(Green Giant):		
In butter sauce	½ cup	120
Harvest Fresh or polybag	½ cup	100
(Larsen) baby	3.3 oz.	130
(Seabrook Farms):		
Baby lima	⅓ pkg.	126
Baby butter bean	⅓ pkg.	139
Fordhooks	⅓ pkg.	98
BEAN, PINK, canned		
(Goya)	½ cup	115

Food and Description	Measure or Quantity	Calories
BEAN, PINTO:		
Canned, regular pack, solids & liq.:		
(Gebhardt)	⅓ of 15-oz. can	245
(Goya)	½ cup (4 oz.)	100
Frozen (McKenzie)	3.2-oz. serving	160
BEAN, RED, canned		
(Goya)	½ cup	79
BEAN, REFRIED, canned:		
(Gebhardt) regular	4 oz.	130
Little Pancho, & green chili	½ cup	80
Old El Paso:		
Plain	4 oz.	106
With sausage	4 oz.	224
(Rosarita):		
Regular	4 oz.	130
With green chilis	4 oz.	120
BEAN, ROMAN,		
canned (Goya)	½ cup	81
BEAN SALAD, canned		
(Green Giant)	¼-oz. serving	80
BEANS 'N FIXIN'S, canned (Hunt's)		
Big John's:		
Beans	3 oz.	100
Fixin's	1 oz.	50
BEAN SOUP (See SOUP, Bean)		
BEAN SPROUT:		
Mung, raw	½ lb.	80
Mung, boiled, drained	¼ lb.	32
Soy, raw	½ lb.	104
Soy, boiled, drained	¼ lb.	43
Canned (Chun King)	4 oz.	40
BEAN, WHITE, canned		
(Goya) solids & liq.	½ cup	105
BEAN, YELLOW OR WAX:		
Boiled, 1″ pieces, drained	½ cup	18
Canned, regular pack, solids & liq.:		
(Del Monte) cut or french	½ cup	18
(Larsen) *Freshlike*	½ cup	25
(Libby's) cut	4 oz.	23
(Stokley-Van Camp)	½ cup	23
Canned, dietetic (Featherweight)		
cut, solids & liq.	½ cup	25
Frozen (Frosty Acres)	3 oz.	25
BEEF, choice grade, medium done:		
Brisket, braised:		
Lean & fat	3 oz.	350
Lean only	3 oz.	189
Chuck, pot roast:		
Lean & fat	3 oz.	278

10

Food and Description	Measure or Quantity	Calories
Lean only	3 oz.	182
Fat, separable, cooked	1 oz.	207
Filet mignon (See STEAK, sirloin, lean)		
Flank, braised, 100% lean	3 oz.	167
Ground:		
Regular, raw	½ cup	303
Regular, broiled	3 oz.	243
Lean, broiled	3 oz.	186
Rib:		
Roasted, lean & fat	3 oz.	374
Lean only	3 oz.	205
Round:		
Broiled, lean & fat	3 oz.	222
Lean only	3 oz.	161
Rump:		
Broiled, lean & fat	3 oz.	295
Lean only	3 oz.	177
Steak, club, broiled:		
One 8-oz. steak (weighed without bone before cooking) will give you:		
Lean & fat	5.9 oz.	754
Lean only	3.4 oz.	234
Steak, porterhouse, broiled:		
One 16-oz. steak (weighed with bone before cooking) will give you:		
Lean & fat	10.2 oz.	1339
Lean only	5.9 oz.	372
Steak, ribeye, broiled:		
One 10-oz. steak (weighed without bone before cooking) will give you:		
Lean & fat	7.3 oz.	911
Lean only	3.8 oz.	258
Steak, sirloin, double-bone, broiled:		
One 16-oz. steak (weighed with bone before cooking) will give you:		
Lean & fat	8.9 oz.	1028
Lean only	5.9 oz.	359
One 12-oz. steak (weighed with bone before cooking) will give you:		
Lean & fat	6.6 oz.	767
Lean only	4.4 oz.	268
Steak, T-bone, broiled:		
One 16-oz. steak (weighed with bone before cooking) will give you:		
Lean & fat	9.8 oz.	1315

Food and Description	Measure or Quantity	Calories
Lean only	5.5 oz.	348
BEEF BOUILLON:		
(Herb-Ox):		
Cube	1 cube	6
Packet	1 packet	8
Lite-Line (Borden) instant, low sodium	1 tsp.	12
(MBT)	1 packet	14
(Wyler's)	1 cube	6
Low sodium (Featherweight)	1 tsp.	18
BEEF, CHIPPED:		
Cooked, home recipe	½ cup	188
Frozen, creamed:		
(Banquet) creamed, *Entree for One*	4-oz. pkg.	90
(Stouffer's)	5½-oz. serving	231
BEEF DINNER or **ENTREE,** frozen:		
(Armour):		
Classic Lites, Steak Diane	10-oz. meal	290
Dinner Classics, Burgundy	10½-oz. dinner	330
(Banquet):		
American Favorites, chopped	11-oz. dinner	434
Extra Helping, regular	16-oz. dinner	864
(Blue Star) *Dining Light,* teriyaki	8⅝-oz. dinner	230
(Conagra) *Light & Elegant,* Julienne	8½-oz. entree	260
(Green Giant)		
Baked, boneless ribs in BBQ sauce with corn on the cob	1 meal	390
Twin pouch, burgundy, with rice & carrots	1 meal	280
(Le Menu):		
Chopped sirloin	11½-oz. dinner	390
Yankee pot roast	11-oz. dinner	360
(Morton):		
Regular	11-oz. dinner	272
Light, sliced	11-oz. dinner	260
(Stouffer's) *Lean Cuisine,* Oriental	8⅝-oz. pkg.	280
(Swanson):		
Regular, 4-compartment, chopped sirloin	11½-oz. dinner	350
Hungry Man:		
Chopped	17¼-oz. dinner	600
Sliced	12¼-oz. entree	330
(Weight Watchers):		
Beefsteak, 2-compartment meal	8¹⁵⁄₁₆-oz. pkg.	320
Oriental	10-oz. meal	260
BEEF, DRIED, canned:		
(Hormel)	1 oz.	45

Food and Description	Measure or Quantity	Calories
(Swift)	1 oz.	47
BEEF GOULASH (Hormel)		
Short Orders	7½-oz. can	230
BEEF, GROUND, SEASONING MIX:		
*(Durkee):		
Regular	1 cup	653
With onion	1 cup	659
(French's) with onion	1⅛-oz. pkg.	100
BEEF HASH, ROAST:		
Canned, *Mary Kitchen* (Hormel):		
Regular	7½-oz. serving	350
Short Orders	7½-oz. can	360
Frozen (Stouffer's)	½ of 11½-oz. pkg.	265
BEEF, PACKAGED		
(Carl Buddig)	1 oz.	38
BEEF, PEPPER ORIENTAL, frozen		
(La Choy) dinner	12-oz. dinner	250
BEEF PIE, frozen:		
(Banquet)	8-oz. pie	449
(Morton)	8-oz. pie	320
(Swanson):		
Regular	8-oz. pie	400
Chunky	10-oz. pie	530
BEEF PUFFS, frozen (Durkee)	1 piece	47
BEEF ROLL (Hormel) Lumberjack	1 oz.	101
BEEF, SHORT RIBS, frozen:		
(Armour) *Dinner Classics,* boneless	10½-oz. dinner	460
(Stouffer's) boneless, with vegetable gravy	½ of 11½-oz. pkg.	350
BEEF SOUP (See SOUP, Beef)		
BEEF SPREAD, ROAST, canned		
(Underwood)	½ of 4¾-oz. can	140
BEEF STEAK, BREADED (Hormel) frozen	4-oz. serving	370
BEEF STEW:		
Home recipe, made with lean beef chuck	1 cup	218
Canned, regular pack:		
Dinty Moore (Hormel):		
Regular	8-oz. serving	210
Short Orders	7½-oz. can	150
(Libby's)	7½-oz serving	160
Canned, dietetic (Estee)	7½-oz. serving	210
Frozen:		
(Banquet) *Buffet Supper*	2-lb. pkg.	1016
(Green Giant):		
Boil'N Bag	9-oz. entree	180

Food and Description	Measure or Quantity	Calories
Twin pouch, with noodles	9-oz. entree	333
(Stouffer's)	10-oz. serving	305
BEEF STEW SEASONING MIX:		
*(Durkee)	1 cup	379
(French's)	1 pkg.	150
BEEF STOCK BASE (French's)	1 tsp.	8
BEEF STROGANOFF, frozen:		
(Armour) *Dinner Classics*	11¼-oz. dinner	370
(Conagra) *Light & Elegant*	9-oz. entree	260
(Le Menu)	9¼ oz. dinner	430
(Stouffer's) with parsley noodles	9¾ oz.	390
*BEEF STROGANOFF SEASONING MIX (Durkee)	1 cup	820
BEER & ALE:		
Regular:		
Black Horse Ale	8 fl. oz.	108
Black Label (Heilemann)	8 fl. oz.	91
Blatz (Heilemann)	8 fl. oz.	93
Budweiser: Busch Bavarian	8 fl. oz.	100
Michelob	8 fl. oz.	113
Old Milwaukee	8 fl. oz.	95
Pearl Premium	8 fl. oz.	99
Schlitz	8 fl. oz.	100
Stroh Bohemian	8 fl. oz.	84
Light or low carbohydrate:		
Budweiser Light; Natural light	8 fl. oz.	75
Gablinger's	8 fl. oz.	66
Michelob Light	8 fl. oz.	90
Old Milwaukee	8 fl. oz.	80
Pearl Light	8 fl. oz.	60
Schlitz Light	8 fl. oz.	64
Stroh Light	8 fl. oz.	77
BEER, NEAR:		
Goetz Pale	8 fl. oz.	53
(Metbrew)	8 fl. oz.	49
BEET:		
Boiled, whole	2"-dia. beet	16
Boiled, sliced	½ cup	33
Canned, regular pack, solids & liq.:		
(Blue Boy) Harvard	½ cup	100
(Del Monte)		
Pickled	4 oz.	77
Sliced	4 oz.	29
(Greenwood)		
Harvard	½ cup	70
Pickled	½ cup	110
(Larsen) *Freshlike:*		
Regular	½ cup	40
Pickled	½ cup	100

Food and Description	Measure or Quantity	Calories
(Stokely-Van Camp) pickled	½ cup	95
Canned, dietetic, solids & liq.:		
(Blue Boy) whole	½ cup	39
(Comstock)	½ cup	30
(Featherweight) sliced	½ cup	45
(Larsen) *Fresh-Lite*	½ cup	40
(S&W) *Nutradiet*, sliced	½ cup	35
BEET PUREE, canned (Larsen)	½ cup	45
BENEDICTINE LIQUEUR (Julius Wile)	1½ fl. oz.	168
BERRY, MIXED, DRINK, canned, *Ssips* (Johanna Farms)	8.45-fl.-oz. container	130
BIG H, burger sauce (Hellmann's)	1 T.	71
BIG MAC (See *McDONALD'S*)		
BIG WHEEL (Hostess)	1 piece	170
BISCUIT DOUGH (Pillsbury):		
Baking Powder, *1869 Brand*	1 biscuit	100
Big Country	1 biscuit	95
Big Country, Good 'N Buttery	1 biscuit	100
Buttermilk:		
Regular	1 biscuit	50
Ballard, Oven Ready	1 biscuit	50
Extra Lights	1 biscuit	60
Extra rich, *Hungry Jack*	1 biscuit	65
Fluffy, *Hungry Jack*	1 biscuit	100
Butter Tastin', 1869 Brand	1 biscuit	100
Dinner	1 biscuit	55
Flaky, *Hungry Jack*	1 biscuit	90
Oven Ready, Ballard	1 biscuit	50
BITTERS (Angostura)	1 tsp.	14
BLACKBERRY, fresh, hulled	1 cup	84
BLACKBERRY JELLY:		
Sweetened (Home Brands)	1 T.	14
Dietetic:		
(Diet Delight)	1 T.	12
(Featherweight)	1 T.	16
BLACKBERRY LIQUEUR (Bols)	1 fl. oz.	95
BLACKBERRY PRESERVE OR JAM:		
Sweetened (Smucker's)	1 T.	53
Dietetic:		
(Estee; Louis Sherry)	1 T.	6
(Featherweight)	1 T.	16
(S&W) *Nutradiet*	1 T.	12
BLACKBERRY WINE (Mogen David)	3 fl. oz.	135
BLACK-EYED PEAS:		
Canned:		
(Allen's)	½ cup	100

Food and Description	Measure or Quantity	Calories
(Goya)	½ cup	105
(Trappey's) any style	½ cup	90
Frozen:		
(Birds Eye)	⅓ pkg.	133
(Frosty Acres)	3.3 oz.	130
(McKenzie; Seabrook Farms)	⅓ pkg.	130
(Southland)	⅕ of 16-oz. pkg.	130
BLINTZ, frozen:		
(Empire Kosher):		
Apple	2½ oz.	100
Blueberry & cheese	2½ oz.	110
Potato	2½ oz.	130
(King Kold) cheese	2½ oz.	132
BLOODY MARY MIX:		
Dry (Bar-Tender's)	1 serving	26
Liquid (Sacramento)	5½-fl. oz. can	39
BLUEBERRY, fresh, whole	½ cup	45
BLUEBERRY PIE (See PIE, Blueberry)		
BLUEBERRY PRESERVE OR JAM:		
Sweetened:		
(Home Brands)	1 T.	52
(Smucker's)	1 T.	53
Dietetic (Louis Sherry)	1 T.	6
BLUEFISH, broiled	3½″ × 3″ × ½″ piece	199
BODY BUDDIES, cereal (General Mills):		
Brown sugar & honey	1 cup	110
Natural fruit flavor	¾ cup	110
BOLOGNA:		
(Eckrich):		
Beef:		
Regular, garlic	1 oz.	90
Thick slice	1½-oz. slice	140
German brand	1-oz. slice	80
Meat, regular	1-oz. slice	90
(Hormel):		
Beef	1-oz. slice	85
Meat	1-oz. slice	90
(Ohse):		
Regular	1 oz.	85
15% chicken	1 oz.	90
(Oscar Mayer):		
Beef	.8-oz. slice	73
Beef	1-oz. slice	90
Beef Lebanon	.8-oz. slice	49
Garlic beef	1-oz. slice	89
Meat	1-oz. slice	70

16

Food and Description	Measure or Quantity	Calories
(Swift) *Light & Lean*	1-oz. slice	95
BOLOGNA & CHEESE:		
(Eckrich)	.7-oz. slice	90
(Oscar Mayer)	.8-oz. slice	74
BONITO, canned (Star-Kist):		
Chunk	6½-oz. can	605
Solid	7-oz. can	650
***BOO*BERRY*,** cereal (General Mills)	1 cup	110
BORSCHT, canned:		
Regular:		
(Gold's)	8-oz. serving	72
(Manischewitz)	8-oz. serving	80
(Mother's) old fashioned	8-oz. serving	90
Dietetic or low calorie:		
(Gold's)	8-oz. serving	24
(Manischewitz)	8-oz. serving	20
(Mother's):		
Artificially sweetened	8-oz. serving	29
Unsalted	8-oz. serving	107
(Rokeach):		
Diet	8-oz. serving	15
Unsalted	8-oz. serving	103
BOSCO (See SYRUP)		
BOYSENBERRY JELLY:		
Sweetened (Home Brands)	1 T.	15
Dietetic (S&W) *Nutradiet,* red label	1 T.	12
BRAN:		
Crude	1 oz.	60
Miller's (Elam's)	1 oz.	87
BRAN BREAKFAST CEREAL:		
(Kellogg's):		
All Bran or *Bran Buds*	⅓ cup	70
Cracklin' Oat Bran	½ cup	120
40% bran flakes	¾ cup	90
Raisin	¾ cup	110
(Loma Linda)	1 oz.	90
(Nabisco)	½ cup	70
(Post) 40% bran flakes	⅔ cup	107
(Quaker) *Corn Bran*	⅔ cup	109
(Ralston-Purina):		
Bran Chex	⅔ cup	90
40% bran	¾ cup	100
Raisin	¾ cup	120
BRANDY (See DISTILLED LIQUOR)		
BRANDY, FLAVORED		
(Mr. Boston):		
Apricot	1 fl. oz.	94
Blackberry	1 fl. oz.	92

Food and Description	Measure or Quantity	Calories
Cherry	1 fl. oz.	87
Ginger	1 fl. oz.	72
Peach	1 fl. oz.	94
BRAUNSCHWEIGER:		
(Eckrich) chub	1 oz.	70
(Oscar Mayer) chub	1 oz.	96
(Swift) 8-oz. chub	1 oz.	109
BRAZIL NUT:		
Shelled	4 nuts	114
Roasted (Fisher) salted	1 oz.	193
BREAD:		
Boston Brown	3″ × ¾″ slice	101
Bran'nola (Arnold)	1.3-oz. slice	90
Cinnamon (Pepperidge Farm)	.9-oz. slice	85
Cracked wheat:		
(Pepperidge Farm)	.9-oz. slice	70
(Wonder)	1-oz. slice	70
Crispbread, *Wasa:*		
Rye, lite	.3-oz. slice	30
Sesame	.5-oz. slice	50
Date-nut roll (Dromedary)	1-oz. slice	80
Flatbread, *Ideal:*		
Bran	.2-oz. slice	19
Extra thin	.1-oz. slice	12
Whole grain	.2-oz. slice	19
French:		
Francisco (Arnold)	1-oz. slice	70
(Wonder)	1-oz. slice	71
Garlic (Arnold)	1-oz. slice	80
Hi-Fibre (Monk's)	1-oz. slice	50
Hillbilly	1-oz. slice	70
Hollywood, dark	1-oz. slice	70
Honey bran (Pepperidge Farm)	1-oz. slice	95
Honey wheat berry (Arnold)	1.1-oz. slice	80
Italian (Arnold) *Francisco*	1 slice	70
Multi-grain (Arnold) *Milk & Honey*	1-oz. slice	70
Natural grains (Arnold)	.8-oz. slice	60
Oat (Arnold) *Bran'nola*	1.3-oz. slice	110
Oatmeal (Pepperidge Farm)	.9-oz. slice	70
Pita (see *Sahara*, Thomas')		
Protein (Thomas')	.7-oz. slice	46
Pumpernickel:		
(Arnold)	1-oz. slice	80
(Levy's)	1.1-oz. slice	80
(Pepperidge Farm):		
Regular	1.1-oz. slice	80
Party	.2-oz. slice	17
Raisin:		
(Arnold) tea	.9-oz. slice	70

Food and Description	Measure or Quantity	Calories
(Monk's) & cinnamon	1-oz. slice	70
(Pepperidge Farm)	1 slice	75
(Sun-Maid)	.8-oz. slice	70
Roman Meal	1-oz. slice	70
Rye:		
(Arnold) Jewish	1.1-oz. slice	80
(Levy's) Real	1.1-oz. slice	80
(Pepperidge Farm) family	1.1-oz. slice	85
(Wonder)	1-oz. slice	70
Sahara (Thomas') wheat or white	1-oz. piece	80
Sourdough, *Di Carlo*	1-oz. slice	70
Sunflower & bran (Monk's)	1-oz. slice	70
Wheat (see also Cracked Wheat or Whole Wheat):		
America's Own, cottage	1-oz. slice	70
(Arnold):		
Bran'nola	1.3-oz. slice	80
Less or *Liteway*	.8-oz. slice	40
Milk & Honey	1-oz. slice	80
Fresh Horizons	1-oz. slice	50
Fresh & Natural	1-oz. slice	70
Home Pride	1-oz. slice	70
(Pepperidge Farm) sandwich	.8-oz. slice	55
(Wonder) family	1-oz. slice	70
Wheatberry, *Home Pride,* honey	1-oz. slice	70
White:		
America's Own, cottage	1-oz. slice	70
(Arnold):		
Brick Oven	.8-oz. slice	60
Country	1.3-oz. slice	100
Less	.8-oz. slice	40
Milk & Honey	1-oz. slice	80
Home Pride	1-oz. slice	72
(Monk's)	1-oz. slice	60
(Pepperidge Farm):		
Regular	1.2-oz. slice	75
Toasting	1.2-oz. slice	85
(Wonder) regular	1-oz. slice	70
Whole wheat:		
(Arnold) *Stone Ground*	.8-oz. slice	50
(Monk's)	1-oz. slice	70
(Pepperidge Farm) thin slice	1 slice	65
(Wonder) 100%	1-oz. slice	69
BREAD, CANNED, brown, plain or raisin (B&M)	½" slice	80
BREAD CRUMBS:		
(Contadina) seasoned	½ cup	211
(Pepperidge Farm)	1 oz.	110

Food and Description	Measure or Quantity	Calories
*BREAD DOUGH:		
Frozen:		
(Pepperidge Farm):		
Country rye or white	⅒ loaf	80
Stone ground wheat	⅒ loaf	75
(Rich's):		
French	1/20 loaf	59
Italian	1/20 loaf	60
Refrigerated (Pillsbury):		
French	1″ slice	60
Wheat or white	1″ slice	80
*BREAD MIX:		
Home Hearth:		
French	⅜″ slice	85
Rye or white	⅜″ slice	75
(Pillsbury):		
Banana	1/12 loaf	170
Cherry nut	1/12 loaf	180
BREAD PUDDING, with raisins	½ cup	248
BREAD STICK (Stella D'Oro):		
Plain	1 piece	41
Sesame	1 piece	50
*BREAD STICK DOUGH (Pillsbury)	1 piece	100
*BREAKFAST DRINK (Pillsbury)	1 pouch	290
BREAKFAST SQUARES (General Mills) all flavors	1 bar	190
BROCCOLI:		
Boiled, with stalk	1 stalk (6.3 oz.)	47
Boiled, ½″ pieces	½ cup	20
Frozen:		
(Birds Eye):		
In cheese sauce	5 oz.	120
Chopped, cuts or florets	⅓ pkg.	25
(Frosty Acres)	3.3 oz.	25
(Green Giant):		
Cuts, polybag	½ cup	18
Spears in butter sauce	3⅓ oz.	40
Spears, mini, *Harvest Fresh*	⅛ pkg.	16
(Larsen)	3.3 oz.	25
(Seabrook Farms) chopped or spears	⅓ pkg.	30
(Stouffer's) in cheese sauce	½ of 9-oz. pkg.	130
BROTH & SEASONING:		
(George Washington)	1 packet	5
Maggi	1 T.	22
BRUNSWICK STEW, canned (Hormel) *Short Orders*	7½-oz. can	220
BRUSSELS SPROUT:		
Boiled	3–4 sprouts	28

Food and Description	Measure or Quantity	Calories
Frozen:		
(Birds Eye):		
Regular	⅓ pkg.	35
Baby, with cheese sauce	4½ oz.	110
(Frosty Acres)	3.3 oz.	35
(Green Giant):		
In butter sauce	½ cup	60
Halves in cheese sauce	½ cup	80
BUCKWHEAT, cracked (Pocono)	1 oz.	104
BUC*WHEATS, cereal (General Mills)	1 oz. (¾ cup)	110
BULGUR, canned, seasoned	4 oz.	206
BURGER KING:		
Apple pie	1 serving	305
Breakfast Croissan'wich:		
Bacon	1 serving	355
Ham	1 serving	335
Sausage	1 serving	538
Cheeseburger:		
Regular	1 serving	304
Double:		
Plain	1 serving	464
bacon	1 serving	510
Condiments:		
Ketchup	1 serving on sandwich	11
Mustard	1 serving on sandwich	2
Pickles	1 serving on sandwich	0
Chicken specialty sandwich:		
Plain	1 serving	492
Condiments:		
Lettuce	1 serving on sandwich	2
Mayonnaise	1 serving on sandwich	194
Chicken Tenders	1 piece	34
Coffee, regular	1 serving	2
Danish	1 piece	500
Egg platter, scrambled:		
Bacon	1 serving	68
Croissant	1 serving	187
Eggs	1 serving	119
Hash browns	1 serving	162
Sausage	1 serving	234
French fries	1 regular order	227
French toast sticks	1 serving	499

Food and Description	Measure or Quantity	Calories
Hamburger:		
Plain	1 burger	262
Condiments:		
Ketchup	1 serving on burger	11
Mustard	1 serving on burger	2
Pickles	1 serving on burger	0
Ham & cheese specialty:		
Plain	1 sandwich	365
Condiments:		
Lettuce	1 serving on sandwich	3
Mayonnaise	1 serving on sandwich	97
Tomato	1 serving on sandwich	6
Milk:		
2% low fat	1 serving	121
Whole	1 serving	157
Onion rings	1 serving	274
Orange juice	1 serving	82
Salad dressing:		
Regular:		
Bleu cheese	1 serving	156
House	1 serving	130
1000 Island	1 serving	117
Dietetic, Italian	1 serving	14
Shakes:		
Chocolate	1 shake	320
Strawberry	1 shake	334
Vanilla	1 shake	321
Soft drink:		
Sweetened:		
Pepsi-Cola	1 regular size	159
7UP	1 regular size	144
Diet Pepsi	1 regular size	1
Whaler:		
Plain sandwich	1 sandwich	353
Condiments:		
Lettuce	1 serving on sandwich	1
Tartar sauce	1 serving on sandwich	134
Whopper:		
Regular:		
Plain	1 sandwich	452
With cheese	1 sandwich	535
Condiments:		
Ketchup	1 serving on sandwich	17

Food and Description	Measure or Quantity	Calories
Lettuce	1 serving on sandwich	1
Mayonnaise	1 serving on sandwich	146
Onion	1 serving on sandwich	5
Pickle	1 serving on sandwich	1
Tomato	1 serving on sandwich	6
Junior:		
Plain	1 sandwich	262
With cheese	1 sandwich	305
Condiments:		
Ketchup	1 serving on sandwich	8
Lettuce	1 serving on sandwich	1
Mayonnaise	1 serving on sandwich	48
Pickle	1 serving on sandwich	0
Tomato	1 serving on sandwich	3
BURGUNDY WINE:		
(Louis M. Martini)	3 fl. oz.	60
(Paul Masson)	3 fl. oz.	70
(Taylor)	3 fl. oz.	75
BURGUNDY WINE, SPARKLING:		
(Carlo Rossi)	3 fl. oz.	69
(B&G)	3 fl. oz.	69
(Great Western)	3 fl. oz.	82
(Taylor)	3 fl. oz.	78
BURRITO:		
*Canned (Del Monte)	1 burrito	310
Frozen:		
(Hormel):		
Beef	1 burrito	220
Cheese	1 burrito	250
Hot chili	1 burrito	210
(Swanson) bran & beef	15¼-oz. meal	720
(Van de Kamp's) regular crispy fried	6-oz. serving	365
BURRITO FILLING MIX, canned		
(Del Monte)	½ cup	110
BUTTER:		
Regular:		
(Breakstone)	1 T.	100
(Meadow Gold)	1 tsp.	35

23

Food and Description	Measure or Quantity	Calories
Whipped (Breakstone)	1 T.	67
BUTTERSCOTCH MORSELS (Nestlé)	1 oz.	150
BUTTER SUBSTITUTE, *Butter Buds:*		
Dry or liquid	⅛ oz. dry or 1 oz. liq.	12
Sprinkles	1 tsp.	140

C

Food and Description	Measure or Quantity	Calories
CABBAGE:		
Boiled, until tender, without salt, drained	1 cup	29
Canned, solids & liq.:		
(Comstock) red	½ cup	60
(Greenwood)	½ cup	60
Frozen (Green Giant) stuffed	½ pkg.	220
CABERNET SAUVIGNON:		
(Louis M. Martini)	3 fl. oz.	62
(Paul Masson)	3 fl. oz.	70
***CAFE COMFORT*, 55 proof**	1 fl. oz.	79
CAKE:		
Regular, non-frozen:		
Plain, home recipe, with butter, with boiled white icing	⅑ of 9″ square	401
Angel food, home recipe	¹⁄₁₂ of 8″ cake	108
Caramel, home recipe, with caramel icing	⅑ of 9″ square	322
Chocolate, home recipe, with chocolate icing, 2-layer	¹⁄₁₂ of 9″ cake	365
Crumb (Hostess)	1¼-oz. cake	130
Fruit:		
Home recipe, dark	¹⁄₃₀ of 8″ loaf	57
Home recipe, made with butter	¹⁄₃₀ of 8″ loaf	58
(Holland Honey Cake) unsalted	¹⁄₁₄ of cake	80
Pound, home recipe, traditional, made with butter	3½″ × 3½″ slice	123
Raisin date loaf (Holland Honey Cake) low sodium	¹⁄₁₄ of 13-oz. cake	8
Sponge, home recipe	¹⁄₁₂ of 10″ cake	196
White, home recipe, made with butter, without icing, 2-layer	⅑ of 9″ wide, 3″ high cake	353
Yellow, home recipe, made with butter, without icing, 2-layer	¹⁄₁₉ of cake	351
Frozen:		
Banana (Sara Lee)	⅛ of 13¾-oz. cake	175

Food and Description	Measure or Quantity	Calories
Butterscotch pecan (Pepperidge Farm) layer	⅒ of 17-oz. cake	160
Carrot:		
(Pepperidge Farm)	⅛ of 11¾-oz. cake	140
(Weight Watchers)	3-oz. serving	180
Cheesecake:		
(Morton) *Great Little Desserts:*		
Cherry	6-oz. cake	460
Cream cheese	6-oz. cake	480
Strawberry	6-oz. cake	470
(Rich's) Viennese	1/14 of 42-oz. cake	230
(Sara Lee):		
Blueberry, *For 2*	½ of 11.3-oz. cake	425
Cream cheese:		
Regular	⅓ of 10-oz. cake	281
Strawberry	⅙ of 19-oz. cake	223
Strawberry, *For 2*	½ of 11.3-oz. cake	420
(Weight Watchers):		
Regular	3.9-oz. serving	200
Strawberry	3.9-oz. serving	180
Chocolate:		
(Pepperidge Farm):		
Layer, fudge	⅒ of 17-oz. cake	180
Supreme, regular	¼ of 11½-oz. cake	310
(Sara Lee):		
Regular	⅛ of 13¼-oz. cake	199
German	⅛ of 12¼-oz. cake	173
(Weight Watchers) German	2½ oz.	200
Coconut (Pepperidge Farm) layer	⅒ of 17-oz. cake	180
Coffee (Sara Lee):		
Almond	⅛ of 11¾-oz. cake	165
Apple	⅛ of 15-oz. cake	175
Butter, *For 2*	½ of 6½-oz. cake	356
Streusel, butter	⅛ of 11½-oz. cake	164
Crumb (See ROLL OR BUN, Crumb)		
Devil's food (Pepperidge Farm) layer	⅒ of 17-oz. cake	180
Golden (Pepperidge Farm) layer	⅒ of 17-oz. cake	180
Grand Marnier (Pepperidge Farm)	1½ oz.	160
Lemon coconut (Pepperidge Farm)	¼ of 12¼-oz. cake	280
Orange (Sara Lee)	⅛ of 13¾-oz. cake	179
Pound:		
(Pepperidge Farm) butter	⅒ of 10¾-oz.cake	130

Food and Description	Measure or Quantity	Calories
(Sara Lee):		
Regular	1/10 of 10¾-oz. cake	125
Banana nut	1/10 of 11-oz. cake	117
Chocolate	1/10 of 10¾-oz. cake	122
Spice (Weight Watchers)	3-oz. serving	170
Strawberry cream (Pepperidge Farm) Supreme	1/12 of 12-oz. cake	190
Strawberries'n cream, layer (Sara Lee)	1/8 of 20½-oz. cake	218
Torte (Sara Lee):		
Apples'n cream	1/8 of 21-oz. cake	203
Fudge & nut	1/8 of 15¾-oz. cake	200
Vanilla (Pepperidge Farm) layer	1/10 of 17-oz. cake	180
Walnut, layer (Sara Lee)	1/8 of 18-oz. cake	210
CAKE OR COOKIE ICING		
(Pillsbury):		
All flavors except chocolate	1 T.	70
Chocolate	1 T.	60
CAKE ICING:		
Butter pecan (Betty Crocker) *Creamy Deluxe*	1/12 can	170
Caramel, home recipe	4 oz.	408
Cherry (Betty Crocker) *Creamy Deluxe*	1/12 can	170
Chocolate:		
(Betty Crocker) *Creamy Deluxe:*		
Regular, chip or milk	1/12 can	170
Sour cream	1/12 can	160
(Duncan Hines) regular or milk	1/12 can	163
(Pillsbury) *Frosting Supreme,* fudge, nut or milk	1/12 can	150
Coconut almond (Pillsbury) *Frosting Supreme*	1/12 can	150
Cream cheese:		
(Betty Crocker) *Creamy Deluxe*	1/12 can	170
(Pillsbury) *Frosting Supreme*	1/12 can	160
Double dutch (Pillsbury) *Frosting Supreme*	1/12 can	140
Lemon (Pillsbury) *Frosting Supreme*	1/12 can	160
Orange (Betty Crocker) *Creamy Deluxe*	1/12 can	170
Strawberry (Pillsbury) *Frosting Supreme*	1/12 can	160
Vanilla:		
(Betty Crocker) *Creamy Deluxe*	1/12 can	170
(Duncan Hines)	1/12 can	163
(Pillsbury) *Frosting Supreme,* regular or sour cream	1/12 can	160

Food and Description	Measure or Quantity	Calories
White:		
Home recipe, boiled	4 oz.	358
Home recipe, uncooked	4 oz.	426
(Betty Crocker) *Creamy Deluxe*	1/12 can	160
*CAKE ICING MIX:		
Regular:		
Banana (Betty Crocker) *Chiquita*, creamy	1/12 pkg.	170
Butter Brickle (Betty Crocker) creamy	1/12 pkg.	170
Butter pecan (Betty Crocker) creamy	1/12 pkg.	170
Cherry (Betty Crocker) creamy	1/12 pkg.	170
Chocolate:		
Home recipe, fudge	1/2 cup	586
(Betty Crocker) creamy:		
Fluffy, almond fudge	1/12 pkg.	180
Fudge, creamy, dark or milk	1/12 pkg.	170
(Pillsbury) *Frost It Hot*	1/8 pkg.	50
Coconut almond (Pillsbury)	1/12 pkg.	160
Coconut pecan:		
(Betty Crocker) creamy	1/12 pkg.	140
(Pillsbury)	1/12 pkg.	150
Cream cheese & nut (Betty Crocker) creamy	1/12 pkg.	150
Lemon (Betty Crocker) *Sunkist*, creamy	1/12 pkg.	170
White:		
(Betty Crocker) fluffy	1/12 pkg.	60
(Betty Crocker) sour cream, creamy	1/12 pkg.	180
(Pillsbury) fluffy:		
Regular	1/12 pkg.	60
Frost It Hot	1/8 pkg.	50
Dietetic (Pritikin) *Frostlite*	1/12 pkg.	25
CAKE MEAL (Manischewitz)	1/2 cup	286
CAKE MIX:		
Regular:		
*Apple (Pillsbury) *Streusel Swirl*	1/16 of cake	260
Angel Food:		
(Betty Crocker):		
Chocolate or one-step	1/12 pkg.	140
Traditional	1/12 pkg.	130
(Duncan Hines)	1/12 pkg.	124
Applesauce raisin (Betty Crocker) *Snackin' Cake*	1/9 pkg.	180
*Banana:		
(Betty Crocker) *Supermoist*	1/12 of cake	260
(Pillsbury) *Pillsbury Plus*	1/12 of cake	250

Food and Description	Measure or Quantity	Calories
*Banana walnut (Betty Crocker)		
Snackin' Cake	⅑ of cake	90
*Boston cream (Pillsbury) *Bundt*	1/16 of cake	270
*Butter (Pillsbury) *Pillsbury Plus*	1/12 of cake	260
*Butter Brickle (Betty Crocker)		
Supermoist	1/12 of cake	260
*Butter pecan (Betty Crocker)		
Supermoist	1/12 of cake	250
*Carrot (Betty Crocker)		
Supermoist	1/12 of cake	260
*Carrot'n spice (Pillsbury)		
Pillsbury Plus	1/12 of cake	260
*Cheesecake:		
(Jell-O)	⅛ of 8″ cake	283
(Royal) No Bake:		
Lite	⅛ of cake	210
Real	⅛ of cake	280
*Cherry chip (Betty Crocker)		
Supermoist	1/12 of cake	180
Chocolate:		
(Betty Crocker):		
*Pudding	⅙ of cake	230
Snackin' Cake:		
Almond	⅑ pkg.	200
Fudge Chip	⅑ pkg.	190
Stir 'N Frost:		
With chocolate frosting	⅙ pkg.	220
Fudge, with vanilla frosting	⅙ pkg.	220
(Duncan Hines):		
Deluxe	1/12 of cake	260
Devil's food	1/12 of cake	280
*(Pillsbury):		
Microwave:		
With chocolate frosting	⅛ of cake	300
Supreme, double	⅛ of cake	330
Tunnel of Fudge	⅛ of cake	290
Pillsbury Plus, chip	1/12 of cake	270
*Cinnamon (Pillsbury)		
Streusel Swirl	1/16 of cake	240
Coconut pecan (Betty Crocker)		
Snackin' Cake	⅑ pkg.	190
Coffee cake:		
*(Aunt Jemima)	⅛ of cake	170
*(Pillsbury) Apple cinnamon	⅛ of cake	240
Date nut (Betty Crocker)		
Snackin' Cake	⅑ pkg.	190
*(Pillsbury):		
Bundt:		
Fudge nut crown	1/16 of cake	220

Food and Description	Measure or Quantity	Calories
Fudge, tunnel	1/16 of cake	270
Macaroon	1/16 of cake	250
Pillsbury Plus:		
Fudge, dark	1/12 of cake	260
Fudge, marble	1/12 of cake	270
Streusel Swirl, German	1/16 of cake	260
Devil's food:		
*(Betty Crocker) *Supermoist*	1/12 of cake	260
(Duncan Hines) deluxe	1/12 pkg.	190
*(Pillsbury) *Pillsbury Plus*	1/12 of cake	270
Fudge (See Chocolate)		
Golden chocolate chip		
(Betty Crocker) *Snackin' Cake*	1/9 pkg.	190
Lemon:		
(Betty Crocker):		
*Chiffon	1/12 of cake	190
Stir 'N Frost, with lemon		
frosting	1/12 pkg.	230
Supermoist	1/12 cake	260
*(Pillsbury):		
Bundt, tunnel of	1/16 cake	270
Streusel Swirl	1/16 cake	270
*Lemon blueberry (Pillsbury)		
Bundt	1/16 cake	200
*Marble (Betty Crocker) *Supermoist*	1/12 cake	260
*Orange (Betty Crocker)		
Supermoist	1/12 cake	260
Pound:		
*(Betty Crocker) golden	1/12 cake	200
*(Dromedary)	1/2" slice	150
Spice (Betty Crocker):		
Snackin' Cake, raisin	1/9 pkg.	180
Supermoist	1/12 cake	260
Strawberry:		
*(Betty Crocker) *Supermoist*	1/12 cake	260
*(Pillsbury) *Pillsbury Plus*	1/12 cake	260
*Upside down (Betty Crocker)		
pineapple	1/9 cake	270
White:		
*(Betty Crocker):		
Stir 'N Frost, with		
chocolate frosting	1/6 cake	220
Supermoist	1/12 cake	230
(Duncan Hines) deluxe	1/12 pkg.	188
Yellow:		
*(Betty Crocker) *Supermoist*	1/12 cake	260
(Duncan Hines) deluxe	1/12 pkg.	188
*(Pillsbury) *Pillsbury Plus*	1/12 cake	260

Food and Description	Measure or Quantity	Calories
*Dietetic:		
(Estee)	1/10 of cake	100
(Pritikin) *Batterlite*, unfrosted	1/10 of cake	90
CAMPARI, 45 proof	1 fl. oz.	66
CANDY, REGULAR:		
Almond, Jordan (Banner)	1¼-oz. box	154
Almond Joy (Peter Paul Cadbury)	1.5-oz. bar	220
Apricot Delight (Sahadi)	1 oz.	100
Baby Ruth	2-oz. piece	260
Bar None (Hershey's)	1½ oz.	240
Bonkers! any flavor	1 piece	20
Breath Savers (Life Savers)	1 piece	8
Butterfinger	2-oz. bar	260
Butternut (Hollywood Brands)	2¼-oz. bar	310
Caramel:		
Caramel Flipper (Wayne)	1 oz.	128
Caramel Nip (Pearson)	1 piece	30
Charleston Chew	2-oz. piece	240
Cherry, chocolate-covered (*Welch's*) dark	1 piece	90
Chocolate bar:		
Brazil nut (Cadbury's)	2 oz.	310
Caramello (Cadbury's)	2 oz.	280
Crunch (Nestlé)	1 1/16-oz. bar	160
Hazelnut (Cadbury's)	2 oz.	310
Milk:		
(Cadbury's)	2 oz.	300
(Hershey's)	1.65-oz. bar	250
(Nestlé)	.35-oz. bar	53
(Nestlé)	1 1/16-oz. bar	159
Special Dark (Hershey's)	1.45-oz. bar	220
Chocolate bar with almonds:		
(Cadbury's)	2 oz.	310
(Hershey's) milk	1.55-oz. bar	250
(Nestlé)	1 oz.	160
Chocolate Parfait (Pearson)	1 piece	30
Chocolate, Petite (Andes)	1 piece	26
Chuckles	1 oz.	92
Clark Bar	1.5-oz. bar	201
Coffee Nip (Pearson)	1 piece	30
Coffioca Parfait (Pearson)	1 piece	30
Creme de Menthe (Andes)	1 piece	25
Crispy Bar (Clark)	1¼-oz. bar	187
Crows (Mason)	1 piece	11
Dutch Treat Bar (Clark)	1 1/16-oz. bar	160
Eggs (Peter Paul Cadbury) creme	1 oz.	136
5th Avenue (Hershey's)	1.93-oz. bar	270
Fudge (Nabisco) bar	1 piece	85

31

Food and Description	Measure or Quantity	Calories
Good Stuff (Nab)	1.8-oz. piece	250
Halvah (Sahadi) original and marble	1 oz.	150
Hard (Jolly Rancher):		
All flavors except butterscotch	1 piece	23
Butterscotch	1 piece	25
Hollywood	1½-oz. bar	185
Jelly bean, *Chuckles*	.5 oz.	55
Jelly rings, *Chuckles*	1 piece	37
Jujubes, Chuckles	.5 oz.	55
Ju Jus:		
Assorted	1 piece	7
Coins or raspberries	1 piece	15
Kisses (Hershey's)	1 piece	24
Kit Kat	1.6-oz. bar	250
Krackel Bar	.35-oz. bar	52
Krackel Bar	1.6-oz. bar	250
Licorice:		
(Switzer) bars, bites or stix:		
Black	1 oz.	94
Cherry or strawberry	1 oz.	98
Chocolate	1 oz.	97
Twist:		
Black (American Licorice Co.)	1 piece	27
Black (Curtiss)	1 piece	27
Red (American Licorice Co.)	1 piece	33
Life Savers	1 piece	10
Lollipops (Life Savers)	1 pop	45
Mallo Cup (Boyer)	9/16-oz. piece	54
Malted milk balls (Brach's)	1 piece	9
Mars Bar (M&M/Mars)	1.7-oz. bar	240
Marshmallow (Campfire)	1 oz.	111
Mary Jane (Miller):		
Small size	1.4 oz.	19
Large size	1½-oz. bar	110
Milk Duds (Clark)	¾-oz. box	89
Milk Shake (Hollywood Brands)	2.4-oz. bar	300
Milky Way (M&M/Mars)	2.24-oz. bar	290
Mint or peppermint:		
After dinner (Richardson):		
Jelly center	1 oz.	104
Regular	1 oz.	109
Chocolate covered (Richardson)	1 oz.	106
Junior mint pattie (Nabisco)	1 piece	10
Mint Parfait (Andes)	1 piece	27
Peppermint Pattie (Nabisco)	1 piece	55
York, pattie (Peter Paul Cadbury)	1¼-oz. serving	160
M & M's:		
Peanut	1.83-oz. pkg.	270

Food and Description	Measure or Quantity	Calories
Plain	1.69-oz. pkg.	240
Mounds (Peter Paul Cadbury)	1.65-oz. serving	230
Mr. Goodbar (Hershey's)	1.8-oz. bar	300
Munch Bar (M&M/Mars)	1.42-oz. bar	220
My Buddy (Tom's)	1.8-oz. piece	250
Naturally Nut & Fruit Bar (Planters) almond/apricot	1 oz.	140
$100,000 Bar (Nestlé)	1¼-oz. bar	175
Orange slices, *Chuckles*	1 oz.	110
Park Avenue (Tom's)	1.8-oz. bar	230
Payday (Hollywood Brands) regular	1.9-oz. bar	250
Peanut bar (Planters)	1.6 oz.	240
Peanut, chocolate-covered:		
(Curtiss)	1 piece	5
(Nabisco)	1 piece	11
Peanut butter cup:		
(Boyer)	1.5-oz. pkg.	148
(Reese's)	.9-oz. cup	140
Peanut Butter Pals (Tom's)	1.3-oz. serving	200
Peanut crunch bar (Sahadi)	¾-oz. bar	110
Peanut Parfait (Andes)	1 piece	28
Peanut Plank (Tom's)	1.7-oz. piece	230
Peanut Roll (Tom's)	1.75-oz. piece	230
Powerhouse (Peter Paul Cadbury)	2 oz.	260
Raisin, chocolate-covered:		
(Nabisco)	1 piece	5
Raisinets (BB)	1 oz.	140
Reese's Pieces (Hershey's)	1.95-oz. pkg.	270
Reggie Bar	2-oz. bar	290
Rolo (Hershey's)	1 piece	30
Royals, mint chocolate (M&M/Mars)	1.52-oz. pkg.	212
Sesame Crunch (Sahadi)	¾-oz. bar	110
Skor (Hershey's)	1.4-oz. bar	220
Snickers	2-oz. bar	290
Spearmint leaves, *Chuckles*	1 oz.	110
Starburst (M&M/Mars)	1-oz. serving	120
Sugar Babies (Nabisco)	1.6-oz. pkg.	180
Sugar Daddy (Nabisco) caramel sucker	1.4-oz. pop	150
Sugar Mama (Nabisco)	¾-oz. pop	90
Summit bar (M&M/Mars)	1 bar	115
Taffy:		
Salt water (Brach's)	1 piece	31
Turkish (Bonomo)	1 oz.	108
3 Musketeers	.8-oz. bar	99
3 Musketeers	2.1-oz. bar	260
Ting-A-Ling (Andes)	1 piece	24

Food and Description	Measure or Quantity	Calories
Tootsie Roll:		
Chocolate	.23-oz. midgee	26
Chocolate	1/16-oz. bar	72
Chocolate	1-oz. bar	115
Flavored	.6-oz. square	19
Pop, all flavors	.49-oz. pop	55
Pop drop, all flavors	4.7-gram piece	19
Twix Cookie bar (M&M/Mars)	1¾-oz. serving	246
Peanut butter cookie bar (M&M/Mars)	1¾-oz. serving	261
Twizzlers	1 oz.	100
Whatchamacallit (Hershey's)	1.8-oz. bar	260
Wispa (Peter Paul Cadbury)	1 oz.	150
World Series Bar	1 oz.	128
Y & S Bites	1 oz.	100
Zagnut Bar (Clark)	.7-oz. bar	85
Zero (Hollywood Brands)	2-oz. bar	210
CANDY, DIETETIC:		
Carob bar, *Joan's Natural:*		
Coconut	3-oz. bar	516
Fruit & nut	3-oz. bar	559
Honey bran	3-oz. bar	487
Peanut	3-oz. bar	521
Chocolate or chocolate-flavored bar:		
(Estee):		
Coconut, fruit & nut or milk	.2-oz. square	30
Crunch	.2-oz. square	22
(Louis Sherry) coffee or orange flavored	.2-oz. square	22
Estee-ets, with peanuts (Estee)	1 piece	7
Gum drops (Estee) any flavor	1 piece	3
Gummy Bears (Estee)	1 piece	5
Hard candy:		
(Estee) assorted fruit	1 piece	11
(Louis Sherry)	1 piece	12
Mint:		
(Estee)	1 piece	4
(Sunkist):		
Mini mint	1 piece	1
Roll mint	1 piece	4
Peanut butter cup (Estee)	1 cup	45
Raisins, chocolate-covered (Estee)	1 piece	5
CANNELLONI, frozen:		
(Blue Star) *Dining Light,* cheese	9-oz. dinner	261
(Celentano)	12-oz. pkg.	380
(Stouffer's) beef & pork with mornay sauce	9⅝-oz. pkg.	240
(Weight Watchers) one-compartment	13-oz. meal	450

Food and Description	Measure or Quantity	Calories
CANTALOUPE, cubed	½ cup (3 oz.)	24
CAPERS (Crosse & Blackwell)	1 tsp.	2
CAP'N CRUNCH, cereal (Quaker):		
Regular	¾ cup	121
Crunchberry	¾ cup	120
Peanut butter	¾ cup	127
CAPOCOLLO (Hormel)	1 oz.	80
CARAWAY SEED (French's)	1 tsp.	8
CARL'S JR. RESTAURANT:		
Bacon	2 strips (10 grams)	50
Cake, chocolate	3.2-oz. piece	380
California Roast Beef 'n Swiss Sandwich	7.2-oz. sandwich	360
Cheese:		
American	.6-oz. slice	63
Swiss	.6-oz. slice	57
Chicken sandwich:		
Charbroiler BBQ	6.3-oz. sandwich	320
Charbroiler Club	8.2-oz. sandwich	510
Cookie, chocolate chip	2¼-oz. piece	330
Danish	3.5-oz. piece	300
Eggs, scrambled	2.4-oz. serving	120
Fish sandwich, filet	7.9-oz. sandwich	550
French toast dips, excluding syrup	4.7-oz. serving	480
Hamburger:		
Plain:		
Famous Star	8.1-oz. serving	590
Happy Star	3.0-oz. serving	220
Old Time Star	5.9-oz. serving	400
Super Star	10.6-oz. serving	770
Cheeseburger, Western Bacon:		
Regular	7½-oz. serving	630
Double	10.4-oz. serving	890
Hot cake, with margarine, excluding syrup	5.5-oz. serving	360
Milk, 2% lowfat	10 fl. oz.	175
Muffins:		
Blueberry	3.5-oz. piece	256
Bran	4-oz. piece	220
English, with margarine	2-oz. piece	180
Onion rings	3.2-oz. order	310
Orange juice, small	8 fl. oz.	94
Potato:		
Baked:		
Bacon & cheese	14.1-oz. serving	650
Broccoli & cheese	14-oz. serving	470
Cheese	14.2-oz. serving	550
Fiesta	15.2-oz. serving	550

Food and Description	Measure or Quantity	Calories
Lite	9.8-oz. serving	250
Sour cream & chive	10.4-oz. serving	350
French fries	Regular order (6 oz.)	360
Hash brown nuggets	3-oz. serving	170
Salad dressing:		
Regular:		
Blue cheese	2-oz. serving	150
House	2-oz. serving	186
1000 Island	2-oz. serving	231
Dietetic, Italian	2-oz. serving	80
Sausage patty	1.5-oz. piece	190
Shake	1 regular size	353
Soft drink:		
Sweetened	1 regular size	243
Dietetic	1 regular size	2
Soup:		
Broccoli, cream of	1 serving	140
Chicken & noodle	1 serving	80
Clam chowder, Boston	1 serving	140
Vegetable, mixed	1 serving	70
Steak Sandwich, *Country Fried*	7.2-oz. serving	610
Sunrise Sandwich:		
Bacon	4.5-oz. serving	370
Sausage	6.1-oz. serving	500
Tea, iced	1 regular drink	2
Zucchini	4.3-oz. serving	300
CARNATION DO-IT-YOURSELF DIET PLAN	2 scoops	110
CARNATION INSTANT BREAKFAST:		
Bar:		
Chocolate chip	1 bar	200
Peanut butter crunch	1 bar	180
Packets, all flavors	1 packet	130
CARROT:		
Raw	5½″ × 1″ piece	21
Boiled, slices	½ cup	24
Canned, regular pack, solids & liq.:		
(Del Monte) sliced or whole	½ cup	30
(Larsen) *Freshlike*	½ cup	30
(Libby's)	½ cup	20
Canned, dietetic pack, solids & liq., (S&W) *Nutradiet,* green label	½ cup	30
Frozen:		
(Birds Eye) whole, baby deluxe	3.3 oz.	40
(Frosty Acres)	3.3 oz.	40
(Green Giant) cuts, in butter sauce	½ cup	80
(Larsen)	3.3 oz.	40

Food and Description	Measure or Quantity	Calories
(Seabrook Farms)	⅓ pkg.	39
CASABA MELON	1-lb. melon	61
CASHEW NUT:		
(Eagle Snacks) honey roast	1 oz.	170
(Fisher):		
Dry roasted	1 oz.	156
Honey, salted	1 oz.	150
Oil roasted	1 oz.	159
(Planters):		
Dry roasted	1 oz.	160
Honey roasted	1 oz.	170
Oil roasted	1 oz.	170
CATFISH, frozen (Mrs. Paul's) breaded & fried, fingers	4 oz.	250
CATSUP:		
Regular:		
(Del Monte)	1 T.	17
(Heinz)	1 T.	18
(Smucker's)	1 T.	21
Dietetic or low calorie:		
(Del Monte) No Salt Added	1 T.	15
(Featherweight)	1 T.	6
(Heinz) lite	1 T.	18
(Hunt's)	1 T.	20
CAULIFLOWER:		
Raw or boiled buds	½ cup	14
Frozen:		
(Birds Eye) regular	3.3 oz.	25
(Frosty Acres)	3.3 oz.	25
(Green Giant) in cheese sauce	½ cup	60
(Larsen)	3.3 oz.	25
CAVATELLI, frozen (Celentano)	⅓ of 16-oz. pkg.	270
CAVIAR:		
Pressed	1 oz.	90
Whole eggs	1 T.	42
CELERY:		
1 large outer stalk	8″ × 1½″ at root end	7
Diced or cut	½ cup	9
(Larsen)	3½ oz.	14
Salt (French's)	1 tsp.	12
Seed (French's)	1 tsp.	11
CERTS	1 piece	6
CERVELAT (Hormel) Viking	1-oz. serving	90
CHABLIS WINE:		
(Almaden) light	3 fl. oz.	42
(Carlo Rossi)	3 fl. oz.	66
(Gallo) white or pink	3 fl. oz.	60
(Louis M. Martini)	3 fl. oz.	59

Food and Description	Measure or Quantity	Calories
(Paul Masson):		
Regular	3 fl. oz.	71
Light	3 fl. oz.	45
CHAMPAGNE:		
(Bollinger)	3 fl. oz.	72
(Great Western):		
Regular	3 fl. oz.	71
Brut	3 fl. oz.	74
Pink	3 fl. oz.	81
(Taylor) dry	3 fl. oz.	78
CHARDONNAY WINE		
(Louis M. Martini)	3 fl. oz.	63
CHARLOTTE RUSSE,		
homemade recipe	4 oz.	324
CHEERIOS, cereal, regular or		
honey & nut	1 oz.	110
CHEESE:		
American or cheddar:		
Cube, natural	1″ cube	68
(Borden)	1 oz.	110
(Dorman's) *Chedda-De Lite*	1 oz.	90
(Kraft):		
American Singles	1 oz.	90
Cheddar	1 oz.	110
Old English	1 oz.	110
Laughing Cow, natural	1 oz.	110
(Polly-O) cheddar, shredded	1 oz.	110
(Sargento):		
Midget, regular or sharp	1 oz.	114
Shredded, non-dairy	1 oz.	90
Wispride	1 oz.	115
Blue:		
(Frigo)	1 oz.	100
(Kraft)	1 oz.	100
(Sargento) cold pack or crumbled	1 oz.	100
Bonbino, *Laughing Cow,* natural	1 oz.	103
Brick (Sargento)	1 oz.	105
Brie (Sargento) *Danish Danko*	1 oz.	80
Burgercheese (Sargento)		
Danish Danko	1 oz.	106
Camembert (Sargento)		
Danish Danko	1 oz.	88
Colby:		
(Featherweight) low sodium	1 oz.	100
(Kraft)	1 oz.	110
(Pauly) low sodium	1 oz.	115
(Sargento) shredded or sliced	1 oz.	112

Food and Description	Measure or Quantity	Calories
Cottage:		
Unflavored:		
(Bison):		
Regular	1 oz.	29
Dietetic	1 oz.	22
(Borden):		
Regular, 4% milkfat	½ cup	120
Lite-Line, 1.5% milkfat	½ cup	90
(Breakstone's) smooth &		
creamy	1 oz.	27
(Dairylea)	1 oz.	30
(Friendship)	1 oz.	30
(Johanna):		
Large or small curd	½ cup	120
No salt added	½ cup	90
(Light n' Lively)	1 oz.	20
(Sealtest)	1 oz.	30
Flavored (Friendship)		
Dutch apple	1 oz.	31
Cream, plain, unwhipped:		
(Frigo)	1 oz.	100
(Kraft) *Philadelphia Brand*:		
Regular	1 oz.	100
Light	1 oz.	60
Edam:		
(House of Gold)	1 oz.	100
(Kaukauna)	1 oz.	100
(Kraft)	1 oz.	90
Laughing Cow	1 oz.	100
Farmers:		
Dutch Garden Brand	1 oz.	100
(Kaukauna)	1 oz.	100
(Sargento)	1 oz.	72
Wispride	1 oz.	100
Feta (Sargento) cups	1 oz.	76
Gjetost (Sargento) Norwegian	1 oz.	118
Gouda:		
(Kaukauna)	1 oz.	100
Laughing Cow	1 oz.	110
(Sargento) baby, caraway		
or smoked	1 oz.	101
Wispride	1 oz.	100
Grated (Polly-O)	1 oz.	130
Gruyère, *Swiss Knight*	1 oz.	100
Havarti (Sargento):		
Creamy	1 oz.	90
Creamy, 60% mild	1 oz.	117
Hoop (Friendship) natural	1 oz.	21
Hot pepper (Sargento)	1 oz.	112

Food and Description	Measure or Quantity	Calories
Jarlsberg (Sargento) Norwegian	1 oz.	100
Kettle Moraine (Sargento)	1 oz.	100
Limburger (Sargento) natural	1 oz.	93
Monterey Jack:		
(Frigo)	1 oz.	100
(Kaukauna)	1 oz.	110
(Sargento) midget, Longhorn, shredded or sliced	1 oz.	106
Mozzarella:		
(Fisher) part skim milk	1 oz.	90
(Kraft)	1 oz.	80
(Polly-O):		
Fior di Latte	1 oz.	80
Part skim milk	1 oz.	80
Smoked	1 oz.	85
Whole milk:		
Regular or shredded	1 oz.	90
Old fashioned, regular	1 oz.	70
(Sargento):		
Bar, rounds, shredded regular or with spices, sliced for pizzas or square	1 oz.	79
Whole milk	1 oz.	100
Muenster:		
(Dorman's)	1 oz.	110
(Kaukauna)	1 oz.	110
(Sargento) red rind	1 oz.	104
Wispride	1 oz.	100
Nibblin Curds (Sargento)	1 oz.	114
Parmesan:		
(Frigo):		
Grated	1 T.	23
Whole	1 oz.	110
(Polly-O) grated	1 oz.	130
(Sargento):		
Grated	1 T.	27
Wedge	1 oz.	110
Pizza (Sargento) shredded or sliced	1 oz.	90
Pot (Sargento) regular, French onion or garlic	1 oz.	30
Provolone:		
(Frigo)	1 oz.	90
Laughing Cow:		
Cube	⅙ oz.	12
Wedge	¾ oz.	55
(Sargento) sliced	1 oz.	100
Ricotta:		
(Frigo) part skim milk	1 oz.	43

Food and Description	Measure or Quantity	Calories
(Polly-O):		
Lite	1 oz.	40
Part skim milk	1 oz.	45
Whole milk	1 oz.	50
(Sargento):		
Part skim milk	1 oz.	39
Whole milk	1 oz.	49
Romano:		
(Polly-O) grated	1 oz.	130
(Sargento) wedge	1 oz.	110
Roquefort, natural	1 oz.	104
Samsoe (Sargento) Danish	1 oz.	79
Scamorze (Frigo)	1 oz.	79
Semisoft, *Laughing Cow:*		
Babybel	1 oz.	90
Bonbel	1 oz.	100
Slim Jack (Dorman's)	1 oz.	90
Stirred curd (Frigo)	1 oz.	110
String (Sargento)	1 oz.	90
Swiss:		
(Dorman's)	1 oz.	100
(Fisher) natural	1 oz.	100
(Frigo) domestic	1 oz.	100
(Sargento) domestic or Finland, sliced	1 oz.	107
Taco (Sargento) shredded	1 oz.	105
Washed curd (Frigo)	1 oz.	110
CHEESE FONDUE, *Swiss Knight*	1 oz.	110
CHEESE FOOD:		
American or cheddar:		
(Borden) *Lite Line*	1 oz.	50
(Fisher) *Ched-O-Mate* or *Sandwich-Mate*	1 oz.	90
(Weight Watchers) colored or white	1-oz. slice	50
Wispride:		
Regular	1 oz.	100
& port wine	1 oz.	100
Cheez-ola (Fisher)	1 oz.	90
Chef's Delight (Fisher)	1 oz.	70
Count Down (Pauly)	1 oz.	40
Cracker snack (Sargento)	1 oz.	90
Garlic & herbs, *Wispride*	1 oz.	90
Jalapeño (Borden) *Lite Line*	1 oz.	50
Loaf, *Count Down* (Pauly)	1 oz.	100
Low sodium (Borden) *Lite Line*	1 oz.	70
Monterey Jack (Borden) *Lite Line*	1 oz.	50
Mun-chee (Pauly)	1 oz.	100
Pimiento (Pauly)	.8-oz. slice	73

Food and Description	Measure or Quantity	Calories
Pizza-Mate (Fisher)	1 oz.	90
Swiss:		
(Borden) *Lite Line*	1 oz.	50
(Kraft) reduced fat	1 oz.	90
CHEESE PUFFS, frozen (Durkee)	1 piece	59
CHEESE SPREAD:		
American or cheddar:		
(Fisher)	1 oz.	80
Laughing Cow	1 oz.	72
(Nabisco) *Easy Cheese*	1 tsp.	16
Blue, *Laughing Cow*	1 oz.	72
Cheese'n Bacon (Nabisco)		
Easy Cheese	1 tsp.	16
Gruyère, *Laughing Cow, La Vache*		
Que Rit, reduced calorie	1 oz.	46
Provolone, *Laughing Cow*	1 oz.	72
Sharp (Pauly)	.8 oz.	77
Swiss, process (Pauly)	.8 oz.	76
Velveeta (Kraft)	1 oz.	80
CHEESE STRAW, frozen (Durkee)	1 piece	29
CHENIN BLANC WINE		
(Louis M. Martini)	3 fl. oz.	62
CHERRY, sweet:		
Fresh, with stems	½ cup	41
Canned, regular pack (Del Monte)		
dark, solids & liq.	½ cup	50
Canned, dietetic, solids & liq.:		
(Diet Delight) with pits,		
water pack	½ cup	70
(Featherweight) dark, water pack	½ cup	60
(Thank You Brand)	½ cup	61
CHERRY, CANDIED	1 oz.	96
CHERRY DRINK:		
Canned:		
(Hi-C)	6 fl. oz.	93
(Lincoln) cherry berry	6 fl. oz.	100
Ssips (Johanna Farms)	8.45-fl.-oz. container	130
*Mix (Hi-C)	6 fl. oz.	72
CHERRY HEERING		
(Hiram Walker)	1 fl. oz.	80
CHERRY JELLY:		
Sweetened (Smucker's)	1 T.	53
Dietetic:		
(Dia-Mel)	1 T.	6
(Featherweight)	1 T.	16
CHERRY LIQUEUR (DeKuyper)	1 fl. oz.	75
CHERRY PRESERVES OR JAM:		
Sweetened (Smucker's)	1 T.	53
Dietetic (Estee)	1 T.	6

Food and Description	Measure or Quantity	Calories
CHESTNUT, fresh, in shell	¼ lb.	220
CHEWING GUM:		
Sweetened:		
Bazooka, bubble	1 slice	18
Beechies	1 piece	6
Beech Nut; Beeman's Big Red;		
Black Jack; Clove; Doublemint;		
Freedent; Juicy Fruit,		
Spearmint (Wrigley's);		
Teaberry	1 stick	10
Bubble Yum	1 piece	25
Extra (Wrigley's)	1 piece	8
Fruit Stripe, regular	1 piece	9
Dentyne	1 piece	4
Hubba Bubba (Wrigley's)	1 piece	23
Dietetic:		
Bubble Yum	1 piece	20
Care Free, regular	1 piece	8
(Clark; *Care*Free*)	1 piece	7
(Estee) bubble or regular	1 piece	5
(Featherweight) bubble or regular	1 piece	4
Orbit (Wrigley's)	1 piece	8
CHEX, cereal (Ralston Purina):		
Corn	1 cup	110
Rice	1 cup	110
Wheat	⅔ cup	110
Wheat & raisins	¾ cup	130
CHIANTI WINE:		
(Italian Swiss Colony)	3 fl. oz.	83
(Louis M. Martini)	3 fl. oz.	90
CHICKEN:		
Broiler, cooked, meat only	3 oz.	116
Fryer, fried, meat & skin	3 oz.	212
Fryer, fried, meat only	3 oz.	178
Fryer, fried, 2½-lb. chicken		
(weighed with bone before		
cooking) will give you:		
Back	1 back	139
Breast	½ breast	160
Leg or drumstick	1 leg	87
Neck	1 neck	127
Rib	1 rib	41
Thigh	1 thigh	122
Wing	1 wing	82
Fried skin	1 oz.	119
Hen & cock:		
Stewed, dark meat only	3 oz.	176
Stewed, diced	½ cup	139
Stewed, light meat only	3 oz.	153

Food and Description	Measure or Quantity	Calories
Stewed, meat & skin	3 oz.	269
Roaster, roasted, dark or light meat, without skin	3 oz.	156
CHICKEN À LA KING:		
Home recipe	1 cup	468
Canned (Swanson)	½ of 10½-oz. can	180
Frozen:		
(Banquet) *Cookin' Bag*	4-oz. pkg.	110
(Blue Star) *Dining Lite,* with rice	9½-oz. entree	290
(Green Giant) twin pouch, with biscuits	9-oz. entree	370
(Le Menu)	10¼-oz. dinner	320
(Stouffer's) with rice	9½-oz. pkg.	330
(Weight Watchers)	9-oz. pkg.	230
CHICKEN, BONED, canned:		
Regular:		
(Hormel) chunk, breast	6¾-oz. serving	350
(Swanson) chunk:		
Mixin' chicken	2½ oz.	130
White	2½ oz.	90
Low sodium (Featherweight)	2½ oz.	154
CHICKEN BOUILLON:		
(Herb-Ox):		
Cube	1 cube	6
Packet	1 packet	12
(Wyler's)	1 cube	8
Low sodium:		
(Featherweight)	1 tsp.	18
Lite-Line (Borden)	1 tsp.	12
CHICKEN, CREAMED, frozen (Stouffer's)	6½ oz.	300
CHICKEN DINNER OR ENTREE:		
Canned:		
(Hunt's) *Minute Gourmet Microwave Entree Maker:*		
Barbecued:		
Without chicken	3.1 oz.	150
*With chicken	6.8 oz.	320
Sweet & sour:		
Without chicken	4.1 oz.	130
*With chicken	7.8 oz.	300
(Swanson) & dumplings	7½ oz.	220
Frozen:		
(Armour):		
Classic Lites:		
Burgundy	11¼-oz.dinner	230
Sweet & sour	11-oz. dinner	250
Dinner Classics:		
Fricassee	11¾-oz. dinner	340

Food and Description	Measure or Quantity	Calories
Milan	11½-oz. dinner	350
(Banquet):		
American Favorites	11-oz. dinner	359
Family Entrees	32-oz. pkg.	1720
(Blue Star) *Dining Lite,* glazed	8½-oz. dinner	243
(Celentano):		
Parmigiana	9-oz. meal	310
Primavera	11½-oz. pkg.	270
(Conagra) *Light & Elegant:*		
Cheese	8¾-oz. entree	293
Parmigiana	8-oz. entree	260
(Green Giant):		
Baked:		
In BBQ sauce with corn on the cob	1 meal	350
Stir fry and garden vegetables	10-oz. entree	250
(La Choy) Fresh and Lite, almond	9¾-oz. entree	290
(Le Menu) sweet & sour	11¼-oz. dinner	450
(Morton):		
Regular:		
Boneless	11-oz. dinner	329
Fried	11-oz. pkg.	431
Light, boneless	11-oz. dinner	250
(Stouffer's):		
Regular:		
Cacciatore, with spaghetti	11¼-oz. meal	313
Divan	8½-oz. serving	336
Lean Cuisine:		
Glazed with vegetable rice	8½-oz. serving	270
& vegetables with vermicelli	12¾-oz. serving	260
(Swanson):		
Regular:		
& dumplings	7½-oz. meal	220
Fried, 4-compartment:		
Barbecue flavor	9¼-oz. dinner	560
Dark meat	10¼-oz. dinner	610
Hungry Man:		
Boneless	17½-oz. dinner	670
Parmigiana	20-oz. dinner	810
(Tyson):		
A l'orange	8¼-oz. meal	300
Français	8¾-oz. meal	350
Parmigiana	11¾-oz. meal	450
(Weight Watchers):		
Cacciatore	10-oz. serving	290
Imperial	9¼-oz. meal	240
Parmigiana	8-oz. serving	290

Food and Description	Measure or Quantity	Calories
CHICKEN, FRIED, frozen:		
(Banquet) assorted	2-lb. pkg.	1625
(Swanson) *Plump & Juicy:*		
Assorted	3¼-oz. serving	270
Breast portions	4½-oz. serving	350
Nibbles	3¼-oz. serving	300
Take-out style	3¼-oz. serving	270
***CHICKEN HELPER** (General Mills):*		
& dumplings	⅕ of pkg.	530
& mushrooms	⅕ of pkg.	470
Teriyaki	⅕ of pkg.	480
CHICKEN & NOODLES, frozen:		
(Green Giant) twin pouch, with vegetables	9-oz. pkg.	365
(Stouffer's):		
Escalloped	5¾-oz. serving	252
Paprikash	10½-oz. serving	391
CHICKEN NUGGETS, frozen		
(Banquet) regular	12-oz. pkg.	932
CHICKEN, PACKAGED:		
(Carl Buddig) smoked	1 oz.	50
(Louis Rich) breast, oven roasted	1-oz. slice	40
CHICKEN PATTY, frozen (Banquet)	12-oz. pkg.	900
CHICKEN PIE, frozen:		
(Banquet) regular	8-oz. pie	450
(Stouffer's)	10-oz. pie	493
(Swanson) regular	8-oz. pie	420
CHICKEN PUFF, frozen (Durkee)	½-oz. piece	49
CHICKEN SALAD (Carnation)	¼ of 7½-oz. can	94
CHICKEN SOUP (See SOUP, Chicken)		
CHICKEN SPREAD:		
(Hormel) regular	1 oz.	60
(Underwood) chunky	½ of 4¾-oz. can	63
CHICKEN STEW, canned:		
Regular:		
(Libby's) with dumplings	8 oz.	194
(Swanson)	7⅜ oz.	170
Dietetic (Dia-Mel)	8-oz. serving	150
CHICKEN STOCK BASE (French's)	1 tsp.	8
CHICK-FIL-A:		
Brownie, fudge, with nuts	2.8-oz. piece	369
Carrot-raisin salad	2.7-oz. serving	116
Chargrill, with bun	5¾-oz. serving	372
Chicken salad:		
Cup	3.4-oz. serving	309
Sandwich	5.7-oz. sandwich	449
Chick-fil-A, with bun	5.7-oz. serving	426
Chick-fil-A Nuggets	8-pack	287

Food and Description	Measure or Quantity	Calories
Coleslaw	3.7-oz. cup	175
Icedream	4.5-oz. serving	134
Pie, lemon	4.1-oz. slice	329
Potato, fries, waffle	3-oz. serving	270
Potato salad	3.8-oz. cup	198
Sandwich	5.4-oz. serving	404
Soup, hearty, breast of chicken:		
Small	8⅓ oz.	131
Large	14.3 oz.	230
CHICK'N QUICK, frozen (Tyson):		
Breast fillet	3 oz.	190
Breast pattie	3 oz.	240
Chick'N Cheddar	3 oz.	260
Cordon bleu	5 oz.	310
Kiev	5 oz.	430
CHICK PEA OR GARBANZO, canned, solids & liq.		
(Allen's; Goya)	½ cup	110
CHILI OR CHILI CON CARNE:		
Canned, regular pack:		
Beans only:		
(Comstock)	½ cup	140
(Hormel)	5 oz.	130
(Van Camp) Mexican style	1 cup	250
With beans:		
(Gebhardt) hot	½ of 15-oz. can	470
(Hormel) regular or hot	7½-oz. serving	310
(Libby's)	7½-oz. serving	270
(*Old El Paso*)	1 cup	349
(Swanson)	7¾-oz. serving	310
Without beans:		
(Gebhardt)	½ of 15-oz. can	410
(Hormel) regular or hot	7½-oz. serving	370
(Libby's)	7½ oz.	390
Canned, dietetic pack:		
(Estee) with beans	8-oz. serving	390
(Featherweight) with beans	7½ oz.	270
Frozen, with beans (Stouffer's)	8¾-oz. pkg.	270
CHILI SAUCE:		
(Del Monte)	¼ cup (2 oz.)	70
(El Molino) green, mild	1 T.	5
(Heinz)	1 T.	17
(Ortega) green, medium	1 oz.	7
(Featherweight) Dietetic	1 T.	8
CHILI SEASONING MIX:		
*(Durkee)	1 cup	465
(French's) *Chili-O*, plain	1¾-oz. pkg.	150
(McCormick)	1.2-oz. pkg.	106
CHOCO-DILE (Hostess)	2-oz. piece	235

Food and Description	Measure or Quantity	Calories
CHOCOLATE, BAKING:		
(Baker's):		
Bitter or unsweetened	1 oz.	180
Semi-sweet, chips	½ cup	207
Sweetened, *German's*	1 oz.	158
(Hershey's):		
Bitter or unsweetened	1 oz.	190
Sweetened:		
Dark chips, regular or mini	1 oz.	151
Milk, chips	1 oz.	150
Semi-sweet, chips	1 oz.	147
(Nestlé):		
Bitter or unsweetened, *Choco-bake*	1-oz. packet	180
Sweet or semi-sweet, morsels	1 oz.	150
CHOCOLATE ICE CREAM		
(See ICE CREAM, Chocolate)		
CHOCOLATE SYRUP		
(See SYRUP, Chocolate)		
CHOP SUEY, frozen (Stouffer's)		
beef with rice	12-oz. pkg.	355
*CHOP SUEY SEASONING MIX		
(Durkee)	1¾ cups	557
CHOWDER (See SOUP, Chowder)		
CHOW MEIN:		
Canned:		
(Chun King) Divider-Pak:		
Beef	¼ of pkg.	91
Chicken	½ of 24-oz pkg.	110
Shrimp	¼ of pkg.	91
(Hormel) Pork, *Short Orders*	7½-oz. can	140
(La Choy):		
Regular:		
Beef	¾ cup	60
Chicken	¾ cup	70
Shrimp	¾ cup	45
*Bi-pack:		
Beef	¾ cup	70
Beef pepper oriental, chicken or shrimp	¾ cup	80
Vegetable	¾ cup	50
Frozen:		
(Armour) *Classic Lites*	10½-oz. meal	220
(Blue Star) *Dining Light,* chicken & rice	11¼-oz. dinner	233
(La Choy):		
Chicken	12-oz. dinner	260
Shrimp	12-oz. dinner	220
(Morton) chicken, light	8-oz. entree	210

Food and Description	Measure or Quantity	Calories
(Stouffer's) *Lean Cuisine,* with rice	11¼-oz. serving	240
CHOW MEIN SEASONING MIX (Kikkoman)	1⅛-oz. pkg.	98
CHURCH'S FRIED CHICKEN:		
Chicken, fried:		
Breast	4.3-oz. piece	278
Leg	2.9-oz. piece	147
Thigh	4.2-oz. piece	306
Wing-breast	4.8-oz. piece	303
Corn, with butter oil	1 ear	237
French fried potatoes	1 regular order	138
CHUTNEY (Major Grey's)	1 T.	53
CINNAMON, GROUND (French's)	1 tsp.	6
CITRUS BERRY BLEND, mix, dietetic (Sunkist)	8 fl. oz.	6
CITRUS COOLER DRINK, canned (Hi-C)	6 fl. oz.	93
CLAM:		
Raw, all kinds, meat only	1 cup (8 oz.)	186
Raw, soft, meat & liq.	1 lb. (weighed in shell)	142
Canned (Doxsee):		
Chopped, minced or whole:		
Solids & liquid	½ cup	97
Drained solids	½ cup	58
Canned (Gorton's) minced, meat only	1 can	140
Frozen:		
(Gorton's) fried strips, crunchy	1 package	480
(Howard Johnson's)	5-oz. pkg.	395
(Mrs. Paul's) fried, light	2½-oz. serving	230
CLAMATO COCKTAIL (Mott's)	6 fl. oz.	80
CLAM JUICE (Snow)	½ cup	15
CLARET WINE:		
(Gold Seal)	3 fl. oz.	82
(Taylor) 12.5% alcohol	3 fl. oz.	72
CLORETS, gum or mint	1 piece	6
COCKTAIL (see individual listings such as **DAIQUIRI, PIÑA COLADA,** etc.)		
COCOA:		
Dry, unsweetened:		
(Hershey's)	1 T.	30
(Sultana)	1 T.	30
Mix, regular:		
(Alba '66) instant, all flavors	1 envelope	60
(Carnation) all flavors	1-oz. pkg.	110
(Hershey's) instant	3 T.	81

Food and Description	Measure or Quantity	Calories
(Ovaltine) hot 'n rich	1 oz.	120
*Swiss Miss, regular or with mini marshmallows	6 fl. oz.	110
Mix, dietetic:		
(Carnation):		
70 Calorie	¾-oz. packet	70
*Sugar free	6 fl. oz.	50
*(Featherweight)	6 fl. oz.	50
Swiss Miss, instant, lite	3 T.	70
COCOA KRISPIES, cereal		
(Kellogg's)	¾ cup	110
COCOA PUFFS, cereal		
(General Mills)	1 oz.	110
COCONUT:		
Fresh, meat only	2″ × 2″ × ½″ piece	156
Grated or shredded, loosely packed	½ cup	225
Dried:		
(Baker's):		
Angel Flake	⅓ cup	118
Cookie	⅓ cup	186
Premium shred	⅓ cup	138
(Durkee) shredded	¼ cup	69
COCONUT, CREAM OF, canned:		
(Coco Lopez)	1 T.	60
(Holland House)	1 oz.	81
COCO WHEATS, cereal	1 T.	44
COD:		
Broiled	3 oz.	145
Frozen:		
(Frionor) Norway Gourmet	4-oz. fillet	70
(Van de Kamp's) Today's Catch	4-oz.	80
COD DINNER OR ENTRÉE, frozen:		
(Armour) Dinner Classics, almondine	12-oz. dinner	360
(Frionor) Norway Gourmet, with dill sauce	4½-oz. fillet	80
COFFEE:		
Regular:		
*Max-Pax; Maxwell House Electra Perk; Yuban, Yuban Electra Matic	6 fl. oz.	2
*Mellow Roast	6 fl.oz.	8
Decaffeinated:		
*Brim, regular or electric perk	6 fl. oz.	2
*Brim, freeze-dried; Decafé; Nescafé	6 fl. oz.	4
*Sanka, regular or electric perk	6 fl. oz.	2
*Instant:		
Maxwell House; Taster's Choice	6 fl. oz.	4

50

Food and Description	Measure or Quantity	Calories
Mellow Roast	6 fl. oz.	8
Sunrise	6 fl. oz.	6
*Mix (General Foods) International Coffee:		
Café Amaretto, Café Français	6 fl. oz.	59
Café Vienna, Orange Cappuccino	6 fl. oz.	65
Suisse Mocha	6 fl. oz.	58
COFFEE CAKE (See CAKE, Coffee)		
COFFEE LIQUEUR (DeKuyper)	1½ fl. oz.	140
COFFEE SOUTHERN	1 fl. oz.	79
COGNAC (See DISTILLED LIQUOR)		
COLA SOFT DRINK (See SOFT DRINK, Cola)		
COLD DUCK WINE (Great Western) pink	3 fl. oz.	92
COLESLAW, solids & liq., made with mayonnaise-type salad dressing	1 cup	119
*COLESLAW MIX** (Libby's)		
Super Slaw	½ cup	240
COLLARDS:		
Leaves, cooked	⅓ pkg.	31
Canned (Allen's) chopped, solids & liq.	½ cup	25
Frozen:		
(Birds Eye) chopped	⅓ pkg.	30
(McKenzie) chopped	⅓ pkg.	25
(Southland) chopped	⅕ of 16-oz. pkg.	25
COMPLETE CEREAL (Elam's)	1 oz.	109
CONCORD WINE:		
(Gold Seal)	3 fl. oz.	125
(Pleasant Valley) red	3 fl. oz.	90
COOKIE, REGULAR:		
Almond Supreme (Pepperidge Farm)	1 piece	70
Animal:		
(Dixie Belle)	1 piece	8
(Nabisco) *Barnum's Animals*	1 piece	12
(Sunshine)	1 piece	8
(Tom's)	½ oz.	62
Apricot Raspberry (Pepperidge Farm)	1 piece	50
Assortment:		
(Nabisco) *Mayfair:*		
Crown creme sandwich	1 piece	53
Fancy shortbread biscuit	1 piece	22
Filigree creme sandwich	1 piece	60
Mayfair creme sandwich	1 piece	65
Tea rose creme	1 piece	53

51

Food and Description	Measure or Quantity	Calories
(Pepperidge Farm):		
Butter	1 piece	55
Champagne	1 piece	32
Chocolate lace & Pirouette	1 piece	37
Seville	1 piece	55
Southport	1 piece	75
Blueberry (Pepperidge Farm)	1 piece	57
Blueberry Newtons (Nabisco)	1 piece	73
Bordeaux (Pepperidge Farm)	1 piece	33
Brown edge wafer (Nabisco)	1 piece	28
Brownie:		
(Hostess)	1.25-oz. piece	157
(Nabisco) *Almost Home*	1¼-oz. piece	160
(Pepperidge Farm) chocolate nut	.4-oz. piece	57
Brussels (Pepperidge Farm)	1 piece	53
Brussels Mint (Pepperidge Farm)	1 piece	67
Butter (Sunshine)	1 piece	30
Cappucino (Pepperidge Farm)	1 piece	53
Chessman (Pepperidge Farm)	1 piece	43
Chocolate & chocolate-covered:		
(Keebler) stripes	1 piece	50
(Nabisco):		
Pinwheel, cake	1 piece	130
Snap	1 piece	19
(Sunshine) nuggets	1 piece	23
Chocolate chip:		
(Keebler) Rich 'n Chips	1 piece	80
(Nabisco):		
Almost Home	1 piece	65
Chips Ahoy!		
Regular	1 piece	47
Chewy	1 piece	65
Snaps	1 piece	22
(Pepperidge Farm):		
Regular	1 piece	50
Chocolate	1 piece	53
Mocha	1 piece	40
(Sunshine):		
Chip-A-Roos	1 piece	60
Chippy Chews	1 piece	50
(Tom's)	1.7-oz. serving	230
Date Nut Granola (Pepperidge Farm)	1 piece	53
Fig bar:		
(Nabisco) *Fig Newtons*	1 piece	50
(Sunshine) Chewies	1 piece	50
(Tom's)	1.8-oz. serving	170
Fruit Stick (Nabisco) *Almost Home*	1 piece	70
Gingerman (Pepperidge Farm)	1 piece	57

Food and Description	Measure or Quantity	Calories
Ginger Snap:		
(Archway)	1 piece	25
(Nabisco)	1 piece	30
(Sunshine)	1 piece	20
Golden Fruit Raisin (Sunshine)	1 piece	70
Hazelnut (Pepperidge Farm)	1 piece	57
Ladyfinger	3¼″ × 1⅜″ × 1⅛″	40
Lido (Pepperidge Farm)	1 piece	95
Macaroon, coconut (Nabisco)	1 piece	95
Mallow Puffs (Sunshine)	1 piece	70
Marshmallow:		
(Nabisco):		
Mallomars	1 piece	65
Puffs, cocoa covered	1 piece	120
Sandwich	1 piece	30
Twirls cakes	1 piece	130
(Planters) banana pie	1 oz.	127
Milano (Pepperidge Farm)	1 piece	60
Mint Milano (Pepperidge Farm)	1 piece	76
Molasses:		
(Archway)	1 piece	100
(Nabisco) *Pantry*	1 piece	65
Molasses Crisp (Pepperidge Farm)	1 piece	33
Nilla wafer (Nabisco)	1 piece	19
Oatmeal:		
(Archway):		
Regular	1 piece	110
Date filled	1 piece	100
(Keebler) old fashioned	1 piece	80
(Nabisco) *Bakers Bonus*	1 piece	65
(Pepperidge Farm):		
Irish	1 piece	47
Raisin	1 piece	57
(Sunshine) Country	1 piece	60
Orange Milano (Pepperidge Farm)	1 piece	76
Orbits (Sunshine)	1 piece	15
Peanut & peanut butter (Nabisco):		
Almost Home	1 piece	70
Nutter Butter, sandwich	1 piece	70
Pecan Sandies (Keebler)	1 piece	80
Raisin:		
(Nabisco) *Almost Home:*		
Fudge chocolate chip	1 piece	65
Iced applesauce	1 piece	70
(Pepperidge Farm) bran	1 piece	53
Raisin Bran (Pepperidge Farm) *Kitchen Hearth*	1 piece	53
Sandwich:		
(Keebler):		
Fudge creme	1 piece	60

Food and Description	Measure or Quantity	Calories
Pitter Patter	1 piece	90
(Nabisco):		
Regular:		
Baronet	1 piece	47
Gaity	1 piece	50
Giggles	1 piece	70
I Screams	1 piece	75
Oreo, regular	1 piece	47
Almost Home	1 piece	140
(Sunshine):		
Regular, Hydrox	1 piece	50
Chips 'n Middles	1 piece	70
Tru Blu	1 piece	80
Shortbread or shortcake:		
(Nabisco):		
Lorna Doone	1 piece	35
Pecan	1 piece	75
(Pepperidge Farm)	1 piece	75
Social Tea, biscuit (Nabisco)	1 piece	22
Sprinkles (Sunshine)	1 piece	70
Sugar cookie (Nabisco) rings,		
Bakers Bonus	1 piece	65
Sugar wafer:		
(Dutch Twin) any flavor	1 piece	36
(Nabisco) Biscos	1 piece	19
(Sunshine)	1 piece	45
Tahiti (Pepperidge Farm)	1 piece	85
Toy (Sunshine)	1 piece	12
Waffle creme (Dutch Twin)	1 piece	45
COOKIE, DIETETIC (Estee):		
Chocolate chip, coconut or		
oatmeal raisin	1 piece	30
Wafer, chocolate covered	1 piece	120
COOKIE CRISP, cereal, any flavor	1 cup	110
*COOKIE DOUGH:		
Refrigerated (Pillsbury):		
Brownie, regular	1 piece	140
Oatmeal Raisin or peanut butter	1 cookie	70
Frozen (Rich's):		
Chocolate chip	1 cookie	138
Oatmeal	1 cookie	125
*COOKIE MIX:		
Regular:		
Brownie:		
(Betty Crocker):		
Fudge, regular size	1/16 pan	150
Walnut, family size	1/24 pan	130
(Pillsbury) fudge:		
Regular	2″ sq. (1/16 pkg.)	150

Food and Description	Measure or Quantity	Calories
Microwave	⅓ of pkg.	190
Ultimate, rocky road	2″ sq. (⅟₁₆ of pkg.)	170
Chocolate chip:		
(Betty Crocker) *Big Batch*	1 cookie	60
(Duncan Hines)	⅟₃₆ pkg.	72
(Nestlé)	1 cookie	60
(Quaker)	1 cookie	75
Fudge chip (Quaker)	1 cookie	75
Macaroon, coconut		
(Betty Crocker)	⅟₂₄ pkg.	80
Oatmeal:		
(Betty Crocker) *Big Batch*	1 cookie	65
(Quaker)	1 cookie	66
Peanut butter (Duncan Hines)	⅟₃₆ pkg.	68
Sugar:		
(Betty Crocker) *Big Batch*	1 cookie	60
(Duncan Hines) golden	1 cookie	59
Dietetic (Estee) brownie	2″ × 2″ sq. cookie	45
COOKING SPRAY, Mazola No Stick	2-second spray	8
CORN:		
Fresh, on the cob, boiled	5″ × 1¾″ ear	70
Canned, regular pack, solids & liq.:		
(Allen's) whole kernel	½ cup	80
(Comstock) whole kernel	½ cup	90
(Del Monte):		
Cream style, golden	½ cup	95
Whole kernel	½ cup	100
(Green Giant):		
Cream style	4¼ oz.	96
Whole kernel, golden	4¼ oz.	79
Whole kernel, *Mexicorn*	3½ oz.	90
(Larsen) *Freshlike*, whole kernel, vacuum pack	½ cup	100
(Libby's) cream style	½ cup	100
(Stokely-Van Camp):		
Cream style	½ cup	105
Whole kernel, solids & liq.	½ cup	74
Canned, dietetic pack, solids & liq.:		
(Del Monte) No Salt Added	½ cup	70
(Diet Delight)	½ cup	60
(Larsen) *Fresh-Lite*	½ cup	80
(S&W) *Nutradiet*, whole kernel, green label	½ cup	80
Frozen:		
(Birds Eye):		
On the cob:		
Farmside	4.4-oz. ear	140
Little Ears	2.3-oz. ear	73
With butter sauce	⅓ pkg.	98

Food and Description	Measure or Quantity	Calories
(Frosty Acres):		
On the cob	1 whole ear	120
Kernels	3.3 oz.	80
(Green Giant):		
On the cob:		
Nibbler	2.7-oz. ear	80
Niblet Ear	4.9-oz. ear	140
Whole kernel, *Harvest Fresh*	½ cup	101
Whole kernel, *Niblets*, golden, polybag	⅓ pkg.	80
(Larsen):		
On the cob	3″ piece (2.2 oz.)	60
Kernels	3.3 oz.	80
(Seabrook Farms):		
On the cob	5″ ear	140
Whole kernel	⅓ pkg.	97
CORNBREAD:		
Home recipe:		
Corn pone	4 oz.	231
Spoon bread	4 oz.	221
*Mix:		
(Aunt Jemima)	⅙ pkg.	220
(Dromedary)	2″ × 2″ piece	130
(Pillsbury) *Ballard*	⅛ of recipe	140
***CORN DOGS,** frozen (Hormel)	1 piece	220
CORNED BEEF:		
Cooked, boneless, medium fat	4-oz. serving	422
Canned, regular pack:		
Dinty Moore (Hormel)	2-oz. serving	130
(Libby's)	⅓ of 7-oz. can	160
Canned, dietetic (Featherweight) loaf	2½-oz. serving	90
Packaged (Carl Buddig) sliced	1-oz. slice	40
CORNED BEEF HASH, canned:		
(Libby's)	⅓ of 24-oz. can	420
Mary Kitchen (Hormel)	7½-oz. serving	360
CORNED BEEF HASH DINNER, frozen (Banquet)	10-oz. dinner	372
CORNED BEEF SPREAD (Underwood)	½ of 4½-oz. can	120
CORN FLAKE CRUMBS (Kellogg's)	¼ cup	110
CORN FLAKES, cereal:		
(General Mills) *Country*	1 cup	110
(Kellogg's) regular	1 cup	110
(Ralston Purina) regular	1 cup	110
CORN MEAL:		
Bolted (Aunt Jemima/Quaker)	3 T.	102

Food and Description	Measure or Quantity	Calories
Degermed	¼ cup	125
Mix, bolted (Aunt Jemima) white	1 cup	392
CORN POPS, cereal		
(Kellogg's)	1 cup	110
CORN PUREE (Larsen)	½ cup	100
CORNSTARCH (Argo; Kingsford's;		
Duryea)	1 tsp.	10
CORN SYRUP (See SYRUP, Corn)		
COUGH DROP:		
(Beech-Nut)	1 drop	10
(Pine Bros.)	1 drop	10
COUNT CHOCULA, cereal		
(General Mills)	1 oz. (1 cup)	110
CRAB:		
Fresh, steamed:		
Whole	½ lb.	101
Meat only	4 oz.	105
Canned, drained	4 oz.	115
Frozen (Wakefield's)	4 oz.	96
CRAB APPLE, flesh only	¼ lb.	71
CRAB APPLE JELLY (Smucker's)	1 T.	53
CRAB AU GRATIN, frozen		
(Gorton's) *Light Recipe*	1 package	280
CRAB, DEVILED, frozen		
(Mrs. Paul's) breaded & fried,		
regular	½ of 6-oz. pkg.	170
CRAB, IMITATION (Louis Kemp)		
Crab Delights, chunks, flakes or legs	2 oz.	60
CRAB IMPERIAL, home recipe	1 cup	323
CRACKERS, PUFFS & CHIPS:		
Arrowroot biscuit (Nabisco)	1 piece	22
Bacon-flavored thins (Nabisco)	1 piece	10
Bacon Nips	1 oz.	147
Bran wafer (Featherweight)	1 piece	13
Bravos (Wise)	1 oz.	150
Bugles (Tom's)	1 oz.	150
Cafe (Sunshine)	1 piece	20
Cheese flavored:		
American Heritage (Sunshine):		
Cheddar	1 piece	16
Parmesan	1 piece	18
Better Blue Thins (Nabisco)	1 piece	7
Cheddar sticks (Flavor Tree)	1 oz.	160
Cheese bites (Tom's)	1½ oz.	200
Cheese Doodles (Wise):		
Crunchy	1 oz.	160
Puffed	1 oz.	150
Chee-Tos:		
Crunchy, regular	1 oz.	150

Food and Description	Measure or Quantity	Calories
Puffed balls or puffs	1 oz.	160
Cheez Balls (Planters)	1 oz.	160
Cheez Curls (Planters)	1 oz.	160
Cheeze-It (Sunshine)	1 piece	6
Corn Cheese (Tom's) crunchy	1⅝ oz.	280
(Dixie Belle)	1 piece	6
Nacho cheese cracker (Keebler)	1 piece	11
Nips (Nabisco)	1 piece	5
Tid-Bit (Nabisco)	1 piece	4
Chicken in a Biskit (Nabisco)	1 piece	10
Chipsters (Nabisco)	1 piece	2
Club cracker (Keebler)	1 piece	15
Corn chips:		
(Bachman) regular or BBQ	1 oz.	150
Dipsy Doodle (Wise)	1 oz.	160
(Featherweight) low sodium	1 oz.	170
(Flavor Tree)	1 oz.	150
Fritos:		
Regular	1 oz.	150
Chili cheese flavor	1 oz.	160
Korkers (Nabisco)	1 piece	8
(Laura Scudder's)	1 oz.	160
(Tom's) regular	1 oz.	155
Creme Wafer Stick (Nabisco)	1 piece	47
Corn Stick (Flavor Tree)	1 oz.	160
Crown Pilot (Nabisco)	1 piece	60
Diggers (Nabisco)	1 piece	4
English Water Biscuit		
(Pepperidge Farm)	1 piece	17
Escort (Nabisco)	1 piece	27
French onion cracker (Nabisco)	1 piece	12
Goldfish (Pepperidge Farm)		
Tiny	1 piece	3
Graham:		
Cinnamon Crisp (Keebler)	1 piece	17
(Dixie Belle) sugar-honey coated	1 piece	15
Flavor Kist (Schulze and Burch)		
sugar-honey coated	1 piece	57
Honey Maid (Nabisco)	1 piece	30
(Rokeach)	8 pieces	120
(Sunshine) cinnamon	1 piece	17
Graham, chocolate or cocoa-covered:		
(Keebler)	1 piece	40
(Nabisco)	1 piece	57
Great Crisps! (Nabisco):		
French onion	1 piece	10
Nacho	1 piece	9
Real bacon or sesame	1 piece	8

58

Food and Description	Measure or Quantity	Calories
Hi Ho (Sunshine)	1 piece	20
Meal Mates (Nabisco)	1 piece	23
Melba Toast (See MELBA TOAST)		
Milk Lunch Biscuit (Keebler)	1 piece	27
Mucho Macho Nacho, Flavor Kist		
(Schulze and Burch)	1 oz.	121
Nachips (Old El Paso)	1 piece	17
Nacho Rings (Tom's)	1 oz.	160
Onion rings (Wise)	1 oz.	130
Oyster:		
(Dixie Belle)	1 piece	4
(Keebler) *Zesta*	1 piece	2
(Nabisco) *Dandy* or *Oysterettes*	1 piece	3
(Sunshine)	1 piece	4
Party (Estee)	½ oz.	70
Party mix (Flavor Tree)	1 oz.	160
Pizza Crunchies (Planters)	1 oz.	160
Ritz (Nabisco)	1 piece	17
Roman Meal Wafer, boxed	1 piece	11
Royal Lunch (Nabisco)	1 piece	60
Rusk, *Holland* (Nabisco)	1 piece	60
Rye toast (Keebler)	1 piece	16
RyKrisp:		
Natural	1 triple cracker	25
Seasoned or sesame	1 triple cracker	30
Saltine:		
(Dixie Belle) regular or unsalted	1 piece	12
Krispy (Sunshine)	1 piece	12
Premium (Nabisco)	1 piece	12
(Rokeach)	1 piece	12
Zesta (Keebler)	1 piece	12
Sea Toast (Keebler)	1 piece	60
Sesame:		
American Heritage (Sunshine)	1 piece	17
Butter flavored (Nabisco)	1 piece	17
Chip (Flavor Tree)	1 oz.	150
Crunch (Flavor Tree)	1 oz.	150
(Estee)	½ oz.	70
Stick (Flavor Tree):		
Regular	1 oz.	150
With bran or low sodium	1 oz.	160
Toast (Keebler)	1 piece	16
Skittle Chips (Nabisco)	1 piece	14
Snackers (Ralston)	1 piece	17
Snackin Crisp (Durkee) *D&C*	1 oz.	155
Snacks Sticks (Pepperidge Farm):		
Cheese	1 piece	17
Lightly salted, pumpernickel, rye & sesame	1 piece	16

Food and Description	Measure or Quantity	Calories
Sociables (Nabisco)	1 piece	12
Sour cream-onion stick		
(Flavor Tree)	1 oz.	150
Spirals (Wise)	1 oz.	160
Table Water Cracker (Carr's) small	1 piece	15
Taco chip (Laura Scudder's)	1 oz.	150
Tortilla chips:		
(Bachman) nacho, taco flavor		
or toasted	1 oz.	140
Doritos:		
Regular	1 oz.	140
Cool Ranch, light	1 oz.	120
Salsa Rio	1 oz.	140
(Laura Scudder's)	1 oz.	140
(Nabisco) regular and nacho	1 piece	11
(Planters)	1 oz.	150
(Tom's)	1½ oz.	210
Tostitos:		
Jalapeño & cheese	1 oz.	150
Traditional	1 oz.	140
Town House Cracker (Keebler)	1 piece	16
Triscuit (Nabisco)	1 piece	20
Tuc (Keebler)	1 piece	23
Twigs (Nabisco)	1 piece	14
Uneeda Biscuit (Nabisco) unsalted	1 piece	20
Unsalted (Featherweight)	2 sections	
	(½ cracker)	30
Waverly (Nabisco)	1 piece	17
Wheat (Pepperidge Farm) cracked		
or hearty	1 piece	25
Wheatmeal Biscuit (Carr's) small	1 piece	42
Wheat Nuts (Flavor Tree)	1 oz.	200
Wheat Snack (Dixie Belle)	1 piece	9
Wheat Snaz (Estee)	1 oz.	110
Wheatsworth (Nabisco)	1 piece	14
Wheat Thins (Nabisco) cheese	1 piece	9
Wheat Toast (Keebler)	1 piece	15
Wheat wafer (Featherweight)		
unsalted	1 piece	13
CRACKER CRUMBS, graham:		
(Nabisco)	2 T.	80
(Sunshine)	½ cup	275
CRACKER MEAL (Nabisco)	2 T.	50
CRANAPPLE JUICE (Ocean Spray)		
canned:		
Regular	6 fl. oz.	129
Dietetic	6 fl. oz.	32
CRANBERRY, fresh (Ocean Spray)	½ cup	26

Food and Description	Measure or Quantity	Calories
CRANBERRY-APPLE JUICE		
COCKTAIL, frozen (Welch's)	6 fl. oz.	120
CRANBERRY JUICE COCKTAIL:		
Canned (Ocean Spray):		
Regular	6 fl. oz.	106
Dietetic	6 fl. oz.	36
*Frozen (Welch's)	6 fl. oz.	100
CRANBERRY-ORANGE RELISH		
(Ocean Spray)	2 oz.	104
CRANBERRY-RASPBERRY		
SAUCE (Ocean Spray) jellied	2 oz.	89
CRANBERRY SAUCE:		
Home recipe, sweetened, unstrained	4 oz.	202
Canned (Ocean Spray):		
Jellied	2 oz.	88
Whole berry	2 oz.	89
CRANGRAPE (Ocean Spray)	6 fl. oz.	108
CRANRASPBERRY (Ocean Spray)	6 fl. oz.	110
CRANTASTIC JUICE DRINK,		
canned (Ocean Spray)	6 fl. oz.	110
CRAZY COW, cereal (General Mills)	1 cup	110
CREAM:		
Half & half (Dairylea)	1 fl. oz.	40
Heavy whipping (Dairylea)	1 fl. oz.	60
Light, table or coffee:		
(Johanna) 18% butterfat	1 T.	30
(Sealtest) 16% butterfat	1 T.	26
Light, whipping, 30% fat (Sealtest)	1 T.	45
Sour:		
(Dairylea)	1 fl. oz.	60
(Johanna)	1 T. (.5 oz.)	31
Sour, imitation (Pet)	1 T.	25
Substitute (See CREAM SUBSTITUTE)		
CREAM PUFFS:		
Home recipe, custard filling	3½" × 2" piece	303
Frozen (Rich's) chocolate	1⅓-oz. piece	146
CREAM OF RICE, cereal	1 oz.	100
CREAMSICLE (Popsicle Industries)	2½-fl.-oz. piece	80
CREAM SUBSTITUTE:		
Coffee Mate (Carnation)	1 tsp.	11
Cremora (Borden)	1 tsp.	12
Dairy Light (Alba)	2.8-oz. envelope	10
N-Rich	3-gram packet	16
(Pet)	1 tsp.	10
CREAM OF WHEAT, cereal:		
Regular	1 oz.	100
*Instant	1 oz.	100

Food and Description	Measure or Quantity	Calories
*Mix'n Eat:		
Regular	1 packet	100
Apple & cinnamon	1 packet	130
Maple & brown sugar	1 packet	130
Quick	1 T.	40
CREME DE BANANA LIQUEUR		
(Mr. Boston)	1 fl. oz.	93
CREME DE CACAO:		
(Hiram Walker)	1 fl. oz.	104
(Mr. Boston):		
Brown	1 fl. oz.	102
White	1 fl. oz.	93
CREME DE CASSIS (Mr. Boston)	1 fl. oz.	85
CREME DE MENTHE:		
(Bols)	1 fl. oz.	122
(Mr. Boston):		
Green	1 fl. oz.	109
White	1 fl. oz.	97
CREME DE NOYAUX (Mr. Boston)	1 fl. oz.	99
CREPE, frozen:		
(Mrs. Paul's):		
Crab	5½-oz. pkg.	248
Shrimp	5½-oz. pkg.	252
(Stouffer's):		
Chicken with mushroom sauce	8¼-oz. pkg.	390
Spinach with cheddar cheese sauce	9½-oz. pkg.	415
CRISP RICE CEREAL:		
(Featherweight) low sodium	1 cup	110
(Ralston Purina)	1 cup	110
CRISPY WHEATS'N RAISINS, cereal (General Mills)	¾ cup	110
CROUTON:		
(Arnold):		
Bavarian or English style	½ oz.	65
French, Italian or Mexican style	½ oz.	66
(Kellogg's) *Croutettes*	⅔ cup	70
(Pepperidge Farm)	.5 oz.	70
C-3PO'S, cereal (Kellogg's)	¾ cup	110
CUCUMBER:		
Eaten with skin	8-oz. cucumber	32
Pared	7½" × 2"	29
Pared,	3 slices (.9 oz.)	4
CUMIN SEED (French's)	1 tsp.	7
CUPCAKE:		
Regular (Hostess):		
Chocolate	1 cupcake	170
Orange	1 cupcake	150
Frozen (Sara Lee) yellow	1 cupcake	190

Food and Description	Measure or Quantity	Calories
*CUPCAKE MIX (Flako)	1 cupcake	150
CUP O'NOODLES (Nissin Foods):		
Beef	2½-oz. serving	343
Beef onion	2½-oz. serving	323
Chicken	2½-oz. serving	343
Chicken, twin pack	1.2-oz. serving	155
Shrimp	2½-oz. serving	336
CURAÇAO:		
(Bols)	1 fl. oz.	105
(Hiram Walker)	1 fl. oz.	96
CURRANT, DRIED (Del Monte)		
Zante	½ cup	204
CURRANT JELLY, sweetened		
(Home Brands)	1 T.	50
CUSTARD:		
Canned (Thank You Brand) egg	½ cup	135
Chilled, Swiss Miss, chocolate		
or egg flavor	4-oz. container	150
*Mix, dietetic (Featherweight)	½ cup	80
C. W. POST, cereal:		
Plain	¼ cup	130
With raisins	¼ cup	120

D

Food and Description	Measure or Quantity	Calories
DAIQUIRI COCKTAIL		
(Mr.Boston):		
Regular	3 fl. oz.	99
Strawberry	3 fl. oz.	111
*DAIQUIRI COCKTAIL MIX:		
*(Bar-Tender's)	3½ fl. oz.	177
(Holland House):		
Instant	.56 oz.	65
Liquid:		
Regular	1 oz.	36
Strawberry	1 oz.	31
DAIRY CRISP, cereal (Pet)	¼ cup	120
DAIRY QUEEN/BRAZIER:		
Banana split	13.5-oz. serving	540
Brownie Delight, hot fudge	9.4-oz. serving	600
Buster Bar	5¼-oz. piece	460
Chicken sandwich	7.8-oz. sandwich	670
Cone:		
Plain, any flavor, regular	5-oz. cone	240
Dipped, chocolate, regular	5½-oz. cone	340
Dilly Bar	3-oz. piece	210
Double Delight	9-oz. serving	490
DQ Sandwich	2.1-oz. sandwich	140
Fish sandwich:		
Plain	6-oz. sandwich	400
With cheese	6¼-oz. sandwich	440
Float	14-oz. serving	410
Freeze, vanilla	12-oz. serving	500
French fries:		
Regular	2½-oz. serving	200
Large	4-oz. serving	320
Frozen dessert	4-oz. serving	180
Hamburger:		
Plain:		
Single	5.2-oz. burger	360
Double	7.4-oz. burger	530
Triple	9.6-oz. burger	710
With cheese:		
Single	5.7-oz. burger	410

Food and Description	Measure or Quantity	Calories
Double	8.4-oz. burger	650
Triple	10.63-oz. burger	820
Hot dog:		
Regular:		
Plain	3.5-oz. serving	280
With cheese	4-oz. serving	330
With chili	4½-oz. serving	320
Super:		
Plain	6.2-oz. serving	520
With cheese	6.9-oz. serving	580
With chili	7.7-oz. serving	570
Malt, chocolate:		
Large	20¾-oz. serving	1060
Regular	14¾-oz. serving	760
Small	10¼-oz. serving	520
Mr. Misty:		
Plain:		
Large	15½-oz. serving	340
Regular	11.64-oz. serving	250
Small	8¼-oz. serving	190
Kiss	3.14-oz. serving	70
Float	14.5-oz. serving	390
Freeze	14.5-oz. serving	500
Onion rings	3-oz. serving	280
Parfait	10-oz. serving	430
Peanut Butter Parfait	10¾-oz. serving	750
Shake, chocolate:		
Large	20¾-oz. serving	990
Regular	14¾-oz. serving	710
Small	10¼-oz. serving	490
Strawberry shortcake	11-oz. serving	540
Sundae, chocolate:		
Large	8¾-oz. serving	440
Regular	6¼-oz. serving	310
Small	3¾-oz. serving	190
Tomato	½ oz.	4
DATE (Dromedary):		
Chopped	¼ cup	130
Pitted	5 dates	100
DE CHAUNAC WINE		
(Great Western) 12% alcohol	3 fl. oz.	71
DELI'S, frozen (Pepperidge Farm):		
Mexican style	4-oz. piece	280
Reuben in rye pastry	4-oz. piece	360
Turkey, ham & cheese	4-oz. piece	270
DESSERT CUPS (Hostess)	¾-oz. piece	62
DILL SEED (French's)	1 tsp.	9
DING DONG (Hostess)	1 cake	172

Food and Description	Measure or Quantity	Calories
DINNER, frozen (See individual listings such as BEEF, CHICKEN, TURKEY, etc.)		
DIP:		
Acapulco (Ortega) with cheddar cheese	1 oz.	64
Avocado (Nalley's)	1 oz.	114
Bacon & horseradish (Kraft)	1 T.	30
Bacon & onion (Nalley's)	1 oz.	113
Barbecue (Nalley's)	1 oz.	114
Blue cheese:		
(Dean) tang	1 oz.	61
(Nalley's)	1 oz.	110
Clam (Nalley's)	1 oz.	101
Cucumber & onion (Breakstone)	1 oz.	50
Guacamole (Nalley's)	1 oz.	114
Jalapeño:		
Fritos	1 oz.	34
(Hain) natural	1 oz.	40
(Wise)	1 T.	12
Onion (Thank You Brand)	1 T.	45
Onion bean (Hain) natural	1 oz.	41
Picante sauce (Wise)	1 T.	6
Taco (Thank You Brand)	1 T.	44
DIP 'UM SAUCE, canned (French's):		
BBQ	1 T.	22
Hot mustard	1 T.	35
Sweet 'n sour	1 T.	40
DISTILLED LIQUOR, any brand:		
80 proof	1 fl. oz.	65
86 proof	1 fl. oz.	70
90 proof	1 fl. oz.	74
94 proof	1 fl. oz.	77
100 proof	1 fl. oz.	83
DONUTZ, cereal (General Mills)	1 cup	120
DOUGHNUT (See also *WINCHELL'S*):		
Regular (Hostess):		
Chocolate coated	1-oz. piece	130
Cinnamon	1-oz. piece	110
Donettes, powdered	1 piece	40
Old fashioned, plain	1.5-oz. piece	180
Powdered	1-oz. piece	110
Frozen (Morton):		
Regular:		
Boston creme	2-oz. piece	180
Chocolate iced	1.5-oz. piece	150
Jelly	1.8-oz. piece	180
Donut Holes	⅓ of 7¾-oz. pkg.	160

Food and Description	Measure or Quantity	Calories
Morning Light, jelly	2.6-oz. piece	250
DRAMBUIE (Hiram Walker)	1 fl. oz.	110
DRUMSTICK, frozen:		
Ice cream, in a cone:		
Topped with peanuts	1 piece	181
Topped with peanuts & cone bisque	1 piece	168
Ice milk, in a cone:		
Topped with peanuts	1 piece	163
Topped with peanuts & cone bisque	1 piece	150
DULCITO, frozen (Hormel) apple	4 oz.	290
DUMPLINGS, canned, dietetic (Dia-Mel)	8-oz. serving	160

E

Food and Description	Measure or Quantity	Calories
ECLAIR:		
Home recipe, with custard filling		
and chocolate icing	4-oz. piece	271
Frozen (Rich's) chocolate	1 piece	234
EEL, smoked, meat only	4 oz.	374
EGG, CHICKEN:		
Raw:		
White only	1 large egg	17
Yolk only	1 large egg	59
Boiled	1 large egg	81
Fried in butter	1 large egg	99
Omelet, mixed with milk &		
cooked in fat	1 large egg	107
Poached	1 large egg	78
Scrambled, mixed with milk &		
cooked in fat	1 large egg	111
EGG DINNER OR ENTREE,		
frozen (Swanson):		
Omelet, Spanish style	7¾-oz. meal	250
Scrambled, with sausage &		
potatoes	6¼-oz. meal	410
*EGG FOO YUNG, dinner:		
(Chun King) stir fry	5 oz.	138
(La Choy)	1 patty plus ¼ cup	
	sauce	125
EGG MIX (Durkee):		
Omelet:		
*With bacon	½ pkg.	310
*Puffy	½ pkg.	302
Scrambled:		
Plain	.8-oz. pkg.	124
With bacon	1.3-oz. pkg.	181
EGG NOG, dairy:		
(Borden)	½ cup	160
(Johanna)	½ cup	195
EGG NOG COCKTAIL		
(Mr. Boston) 15% alcohol	3 fl. oz.	177
EGGPLANT:		
Boiled, drained	4 oz.	22

Food and Description	Measure or Quantity	Calories
Frozen:		
(Buitoni) parmigiana	5 oz.	155
(Celentano) rollettes	11-oz. pkg.	420
(Mrs. Paul's):		
Parmesan	5½-oz. serving	270
Sticks, breaded & fried	3½-oz. serving	240
(Weight Watchers) Parmesan	13-oz. pkg.	285
EGG ROLL, frozen:		
(Chun King):		
Chicken	.65-oz. piece	37
Meat & shrimp	2.6-oz. piece	151
Shrimp	.8-oz. piece	41
(La Choy):		
Almond chicken, entree	2 egg rolls	450
Beef & broccoli, entree	2 egg rolls	380
Chicken	.5-oz. piece	30
Lobster	3-oz. piece	180
Shrimp	.5-oz. piece	27
EGG ROLL DINNER, frozen		
(Van de Kamp's) Cantonese	10½-oz. serving	560
EGG SUBSTITUTE:		
Egg Magic (Featherweight)	½ envelope	60
*Scramblers (Morningstar Farms)	1 egg substitute	35
Second Nature (Avoset)	3 T.	42
ENCHILADA OR ENCHILADA DINNER, frozen:		
Beef:		
(Banquet):		
Dinner	12-oz. meal	497
Entree	2-lb. pkg	1056
(Green Giant) Sonora style	12-oz. entree	700
(Hormel)	1 enchilada	140
(Morton)	11-oz. dinner	280
(Van de Kamp's):		
Dinner, regular	12-oz. dinner	390
Entree, shredded	5½-oz. serving	180
Cheese:		
(Banquet)	12-oz. dinner	543
(Van de Kamp's)	12-oz. dinner	450
Chicken (Van de Kamp's)	7½-oz. pkg.	250
ENCHILADA SAUCE:		
Canned:		
(Del Monte) hot or mild	½ cup	45
(El Molino) hot	1 T.	8
Old El Paso, hot	¼ cup	27
*Mix (Durkee)	½ cup	29
ENDIVE, CURLY OR ESCAROLE, cut	½ cup	7
ESPRESSO COFFEE LIQUEUR	1 fl. oz.	104

F

Food and Description	Measure or Quantity	Calories
FARINA:		
(Hi-O) dry, regular	1 T.	40
Malt-O-Meal, dry:		
Regular	1 oz.	96
Quick cooking	1 oz.	100
*(Pillsbury) made with milk and salt	⅔ cup	200
FAT, COOKING:		
Crisco:		
Regular	1 T.	110
Butter flavor	1 T.	126
(Rokeach) neutral nyafat	1 T.	99
Spry	1 T.	94
FENNEL SEED (French's)	1 tsp.	8
FETTUCINI ALFREDO, frozen (Stouffer's)	½ of 10-oz. pkg.	270
FIG:		
Small	1½" fig	30
Canned, regular pack (Del Monte) whole, solids & liq.	½ cup	100
Dried (Sun-Maid), Calimyrna	½ cup	250
FIG JUICE (Sunsweet)	6 fl. oz.	120
FIGURINES (Pillsbury) all flavors	1 bar	100
FILBERT:		
Shelled	1 oz.	180
(Fisher) oil dipped, salted	½ cup	360
FISH CAKE, frozen (Mrs. Paul's):		
Breaded & fried	2-oz. piece	110
Thins, breaded & fried	½ of 10-oz. pkg.	300
FISH & CHIPS, frozen:		
(Gorton's)	1 pkg.	1350
(Swanson):		
Regular	5½-oz. entree	320
Hungry Man	14¾-oz. dinner	770
(Van de Kamp's) batter dipped, french fried	7-oz. pkg.	440
FISH DINNER, frozen:		
(Banquet)	8¾-oz. dinner	553
(Morton)	10-oz. dinner	320
(Mrs. Paul's) Parmesan	½ of 10-oz. pkg.	220

Food and Description	Measure or Quantity	Calories
(Stouffer's) *Lean Cuisine,* Florentine	9-oz. pkg.	230
(Weight Watchers):		
Au gratin	9½-oz. meal	200
Oven fried	6¾-oz. meal	220
FISH FILLET, frozen:		
(Frionor) *Bunch O' Crunch,* breaded	1 piece	140
(Gorton's):		
Regular, crunchy	1 piece	175
Light Recipe, tempura batter	1 piece	190
(Mrs. Paul's):		
Batter fried, crunchy	2¼-oz. piece	155
Breaded & fried, light & natural	1 piece	290
(Van de Kamp's):		
Batter dipped, french fried	3-oz. piece	180
Country seasoned	2-oz. piece	200
FISH KABOBS, frozen:		
(Mrs. Paul's) light batter	⅓ pkg.	200
(Van de Kamp's) batter dipped, french fried	4-oz. piece	240
FISH NUGGET, frozen (Frionor) *Bunch O' Crunch,* breaded	1 piece	40
FISH SANDWICH, frozen (Frionor) *Bunch O' Crunch,* microwave	5-oz. sandwich	320
FISH SEASONING (Featherweight)	¼ tsp.	<1
FISH STICKS, frozen:		
(Frionor) *Bunch O' Crunch,* breaded	.7-oz. piece	58
(Gorton's) potato crisp	1 piece	60
(Mrs. Paul's):		
Batter fried	1 piece	69
Breaded & fried	1 piece	43
(Van de Kamp's) batter dipped, french fried	1-oz. piece	55
FIT'N FROSTY (Alba '77):		
Chocolate or marshmallow flavor	1 envelope	70
Strawberry	1 envelope	74
Vanilla	1 envelope	69
*****FIVE ALIVE** (Snow Crop)	6 fl. oz.	85
FLOUNDER:		
Baked	4 oz.	229
Frozen:		
(Frionor) *Norway Gourmet*	4-oz. fillet	60
(Gorton's) *Fishmarket Fresh*	4 oz.	90
(Mrs. Paul's) fillets, breaded & fried, crispy, crunchy	2-oz. piece	140
FLOUNDER DINNER OR ENTREE, frozen (Le Menu)	10½-oz. dinner	340

Food and Description	Measure or Quantity	Calories
FLOUR:		
(Aunt Jemima) self-rising	¼ cup	109
Ballard, self-rising	¼ cup	100
Bisquick (Betty Crocker)	¼ cup	120
(Elam's):		
Brown rice, whole grain	¼ cup	146
Buckwheat, pure	¼ cup	92
Pastry	1 oz.	102
Rye, whole grain	¼ cup	89
Soy	1 oz.	98
Gold Medal (Betty Crocker)		
all-purpose or high protein	¼ cup	100
La Pina	¼ cup	100
Pillsbury's Best:		
All-purpose or rye, medium	¼ cup	100
Sauce & gravy	2 T.	50
Self-rising	¼ cup	95
Presto, self-rising	¼ cup	98
Wondra	¼ cup	100
FOOD STICKS (Pillsbury) chocolate	1 piece	45
***FRANKEN*BERRY,** cereal		
(General Mills)	1 cup	110
FRANKFURTER:		
(Eckrich):		
Beef, or meat	1.6-oz. frankfurter	150
Beef or meat, jumbo	2-oz. frankfurter	190
Meat	1.2-oz. frankfurter	120
(Empire Kosher):		
Chicken	2-oz. frankfurter	106
Turkey	2-oz. frankfurter	107
(Hormel):		
Beef	1.6-oz. frankfurter	139
Range Brand, Wrangler, smoked	1 frankfurter	160
(Hygrade) beef, *Ball Park*	2-oz. frankfurter	169
(Louis Rich) turkey	1.5-oz. frankfurter	95
(Ohse):		
Regular, beef	1-oz. frankfurter	85
Wiener:		
Regular	1-oz. frankfurter	90
Chicken	1-oz. frankfurter	85
(Oscar Mayer):		
Bacon & cheddar	1.6-oz. frankfurter	143
Beef	1.6-oz. frankfurter	145
Cheese:		
Regular	1.6-oz. frankfurter	145
Nacho	1.6-oz. frankfurter	138
Little Wiener	2" frankfurter	28
Wiener	1.6-oz. frankfurter	145

Food and Description	Measure or Quantity	Calories
FRANKS-N-BLANKETS, frozen (Durkee)	1 piece	45
FRENCH TOAST, frozen:		
(Aunt Jemima):		
Regular	1 slice	85
Cinnamon swirl	1 slice	97
(Swanson) with sausage, plain	6½-oz. meal	450
FRITTERS, frozen (Mrs. Paul's):		
Apple	2-oz. piece	125
Clam	1.9-oz. piece	131
Corn	2-oz. piece	73
Shrimp	½ of 7¾-oz. pkg.	242
FROOT LOOPS, cereal (Kellogg's)	1 cup	110
FROSTED RICE, cereal (Kellogg's)	1 cup	110
FROSTEE (Borden):		
Chocolate	1 cup	200
Strawberry	1 cup	180
FROSTS (Libby's):		
Dry:		
Banana	.5 oz.	50
Orange, strawberry or pineapple	.5 oz.	60
Liquid:		
Banana	7 fl. oz.	120
Orange or strawberry	8 fl. oz.	120
FROZEN DESSERT, dietetic (See also *TOFUTTI*):		
(Baskin-Robbins):		
Low, Lite 'N Luscious	½ cup (4 fl. oz.)	80–100
Special Diet	1 scoop (2½ fl. oz.)	90
Eskimo, bar, chocolate covered	2½-fl.-oz. bar	110
(SugarLo) all flavors	¼ pt.	135
FRUIT BITS, dried (Sun-Maid)	1 oz.	90
FRUIT COCKTAIL:		
Canned, regular pack, solids & liq.:		
(Del Monte) regular or chunky	½ cup	94
(Libby's)	½ cup	101
(Stokely-Van Camp)	½ cup	95
Canned, dietetic or low calorie, solids & liq.:		
(Del Monte) Lite	½ cup	58
(Diet Delight):		
Syrup pack	½ cup	50
Water pack	½ cup	40
(Featherweight):		
Juice pack	½ cup	50
Water pack	½ cup	40
(Libby's) water pack	½ cup	50
(S&W) *Nutradiet:*		
Juice pack	½ cup	50

Food and Description	Measure or Quantity	Calories
Water pack	½ cup	40
FRUIT COMPOTE (Rokeach)	½ cup	120
FRUIT COUNTRY (Comstock):		
Apple or blueberry	¼ pkg.	160
Cherry	¼ pkg.	180
FRUIT CUP (Del Monte):		
Mixed fruits	5-oz. container	110
Peaches, diced	5-oz. container	116
FRUIT, MIXED:		
Canned (Del Monte) lite, chunky	½ cup	58
Frozen (Birds Eye) quick thaw	5-oz. serving	150
FRUIT & FIBER CEREAL (Post)	½ cup	103
FRUIT JUICE, canned (Sun-Maid)	6 fl. oz.	100
FRUIT 'N APPLE JUICE (Tree Top)	6 fl. oz.	90
FRUIT 'N GRAPE JUICE (Tree Top):		
Canned	6 fl. oz.	100
*Frozen	6 fl. oz.	110
FRUIT 'N JUICE BAR (Dole)	2½-fl.-oz. bar	70
FRUIT & NUT MIX (Carnation):		
All fruit	.9-oz. pouch	80
Deluxe trail mix or raisins & nuts	.9-oz. pouch	130
Tropical fruit & nuts	.9-oz. pouch	100
FRUIT PUNCH:		
Canned:		
Capri Sun	6¾ fl. oz.	102
(Hi-C)	6 fl. oz.	93
(Lincoln)	6 fl. oz.	90
Chilled:		
Five Alive (Snow Crop)	6 fl. oz.	87
(Sunkist)	8.45 fl. oz.	140
*Frozen, *Five Alive* (Snow Crop)	6 fl. oz.	87
*Mix (Hi-C)	6 fl. oz.	72
FRUIT ROLL:		
(Betty Crocker)	1 piece	50
(Flavor Tree)	¾-oz. roll	80
(Sunkist)	½-oz. piece	50
FRUIT SALAD:		
Canned, regular pack:		
(Del Monte) fruits for salad	½ cup	93
(Libby's)	½ cup	99
Canned, dietetic or low calorie:		
(Diet Delight)	½ cup	60
(Featherweight):		
Juice pack	½ cup	50
Water pack	½ cup	40
(S&W) *Nutradiet:*		
Juice pack	½ cup	60

Food and Description	Measure or Quantity	Calories
Water pack	½ cup	35
FRUIT SQUARES, frozen		
(Pepperidge Farm)	2½-oz. piece	230
FUDGSICLE (Popsicle Industries)	2½-fl.-oz. bar	100

G

Food and Description	Measure or Quantity	Calories
GARLIC:		
Flakes (Gilroy)	1 tsp.	5
Powder (French's)	1 tsp.	5
Spread (Lawry's)	1 T.	79
GEFILTE FISH, canned:		
(Mother's):		
Jellied, old world	4-oz. serving	70
Jellied, white fish & pike	4-oz. serving	60
In liquid broth	4-oz. serving	70
(Rokeach):		
Natural Broth	2-oz. serving	46
Old Vienna:		
Regular	2-oz. serving	52
Jelled	2-oz. serving	54
GELATIN, dry, *Carmel Kosher*	7-gram envelope	30
GELATIN DESSERT MIX:		
Regular:		
Carmel Kosher, all flavors	½ cup	80
(Jell-O) all flavors	½ cup	81
Dietetic:		
Carmel Kosher	½ cup	8
(D-Zerta) all flavors	½ cup	6
(Featherweight) artificially		
sweetened or regular	½ cup	10
*(Royal)	½ cup	12
GELATIN, DRINKING (Knox)		
orange	1 envelope	50
GERMAN STYLE DINNER, frozen		
(Swanson)	11¾-oz. dinner	370
GIN, SLOE:		
(Bols)	1 fl. oz.	85
(DeKuyper)	1 fl. oz.	70
(Mr. Boston)	1 fl. oz.	68
GINGER, powder (French's)	1 tsp.	6
GINGERBREAD:		
Home recipe (USDA)	1.9-oz. piece	174
Mix:		
(Betty Crocker)	⅑ of cake	210
(Dromedary)	2″ × 2″ square	100

Food and Description	Measure or Quantity	Calories
(Pillsbury)	3" square	190
GOLDEN GRAHAMS, cereal		
(General Mills)	¾ cup	110
GOOBER GRAPE (Smucker's)	1 T.	90
GOOD HUMOR (See ICE CREAM)		
GOOD N' PUDDIN		
(Popsicle Industries) all flavors	2⅓-fl.-oz. bar	170
GOOSE, roasted, meat & skin	4 oz.	500
GRAHAM CRAKOS, cereal		
(Kellogg's)	1 cup	110
GRAHAM CRAKOS, cereal		
GRANOLA BAR:		
Nature Valley:		
Regular:		
Almond or cinnamon	1 piece	110
Coconut or peanut	1 piece	120
Chewy:		
Apple	1 piece	130
Peanut butter	1 piece	140
New Trail:		
Chocolate chip or peanut butter	1.3-oz. piece	200
Cocoa creme	1.3-oz. piece	90
*GRANOLA BAR MIX, chewy,		
Nature Valley, Bake-A-Bar	1 bar	100
GRANOLA CEREAL:		
Nature Valley:		
Cinnamon & raisin, fruit & nut or		
toasted oat	⅓ cup	130
Coconut & honey	⅓ cup	150
Sun Country:		
With almonds	1 oz.	130
With raisins & dates	1 oz.	130
GRANOLA CLUSTERS,		
Nature Valley:		
Almond	1 piece	140
Caramel & raisin	1 piece	150
GRANOLA & FRUIT BAR,		
Nature Valley	1 bar	150
GRANOLA SNACK:		
Nature Valley	1 pouch	140
Kudos (M&M/Mars):		
Chocolate chip	1¼-oz. piece	180
Peanut butter	1.3-oz. piece	190
Nature Valley	1 piece	140
GRAPE:		
American, ripe (slipskin)	3½" × 3" bunch	43
Canned, dietetic (Featherweight)		
light, seedless, water pack	½ cup	60
GRAPE DRINK:		
Canned:		
Capri Sun	6¾ fl. oz.	104

Food and Description	Measure or Quantity	Calories
(Hi-C)	6 fl. oz.	89
(Lincoln)	6 fl. oz.	90
(Welchade)	6 fl. oz.	90
Chilled (Sunkist)	8.45 fl. oz.	140
*Frozen (Welchade)	6 fl. oz.	90
*Mix:		
Regular (Hi-C)	6 fl. oz.	68
Dietetic (Sunkist)	8 fl. oz.	6
GRAPEFRUIT:		
Pink & red:		
Seeded type	½ med. grapefruit	46
Seedless type	½ med. grapefruit	49
White:		
Seeded type	½ med. grapefruit	44
Seedless type	½ med. grapefruit	46
Canned, regular pack (Del Monte) in syrup	½ cup	74
Canned, dietetic pack, solids & liq.:		
(Del Monte) sections	½ cup	45
(Diet Delight) sections	½ cup	45
(Featherweight) sections, juice pack	½ cup	40
(S&W) *Nutradiet*	½ cup	40
GRAPEFRUIT DRINK, canned (Lincoln)	6 fl. oz.	104
GRAPEFRUIT JUICE:		
Fresh, pink, red or white	½ cup	46
Canned, sweetened:		
(Del Monte)	6 fl. oz.	89
(Texsun)	6 fl. oz.	77
Canned, unsweetened:		
(Del Monte)	6 fl. oz.	72
(Ocean Spray)	6 fl. oz.	64
(Texsun)	6 fl. oz.	77
Chilled (Minute Maid)	6 fl. oz.	75
GRAPEFRUIT JUICE COCKTAIL, canned (Ocean Spray) pink	6 fl. oz.	84
GRAPEFRUIT-ORANGE JUICE COCKTAIL, canned, Musselman's	6 fl. oz.	67
GRAPE JAM (Smucker)	1 T.	53
GRAPE JELLY:		
Sweetened:		
(Smucker's)	1 T.	53
(Welch's)	1 T.	52
Dietetic:		
(Diet Delight)	1 T.	12
(Estee)	1 T.	6
(Welch's)	1 T.	30

Food and Description	Measure or Quantity	Calories
GRAPE JUICE:		
Canned, unsweetened:		
(Seneca Foods)	6 fl. oz.	118
(Tree Top) sparkling	6 fl. oz.	120
(Welch's) regular or red	6 fl. oz.	120
*Frozen:		
(Minute Maid)	6 fl. oz.	99
(Welch's)	6 fl. oz.	100
GRAPE JUICE DRINK, chilled		
(Sunkist)	8.45 fl. oz.	140
GRAPE NUTS, cereal (Post):		
Regular	¼ cup (1 oz.)	110
Flakes	⅞ cup (1 oz.)	100
GRAVY, canned:		
Au jus (Franco-American)	2-oz. serving	5
Beef (Franco-American)	2-oz. serving	25
Brown:		
(Estee) dietetic	¼ cup	14
(Franco-American) with onion	2-oz. serving	25
(Howard Johnson's)	½ cup	51
Ready Gravy	¼ cup	44
Chicken (Franco-American):		
Regular	2-oz. serving	50
Giblet	2-oz. serving	26
Chicken & herb	¼ cup	20
Mushroom (Franco-American)	2-oz. serving	25
Pork (Franco-American)	2-oz. serving	40
Turkey:		
(Franco-American)	2-oz. serving	30
(Howard Johnson's) giblet	½ cup	55
GRAVYMASTER	1 tsp.	11
GRAVY MIX:		
Regular:		
Au jus:		
*(Durkee)	½ cup	15
*(French's) *Gravy Makins*	½ cup	20
Brown:		
*(Durkee) regular	½ cup	29
*(French's) *Gravy Makins*	½ cup	40
*(McCormick)	.85-oz. pkg.	82
*(Pillsbury)	½ cup	30
*(Spatini)	1 oz.	8
Chicken:		
*(Durkee) regular	½ cup	43
*(French's) *Gravy Makins*	½ cup	50
*(Pillsbury)	½ cup	50
Home style:		
*(Durkee)	½ cup	35
*(French's) *Gravy Makins*	½ cup	40

Food and Description	Measure or Quantity	Calories
*(Pillsbury)	½ cup	30
Meatloaf (Durkee) *Roasting Bag*	1.5-oz. pkg.	129
Mushroom:		
*(Durkee)	½ cup	30
*(French's) *Gravy Makins*	½ cup	40
Onion:		
*(Durkee)	½ cup	42
*(French's) *Gravy Makins*	½ cup	50
*(McCormick)	.85-oz. pkg.	72
Pork:		
*(Durkee)	½ cup	35
*(French's) *Gravy Makins*	½ cup	40
*Swiss Steak (Durkee)	½ cup	23
Turkey:		
*(Durkee)	½ cup	47
*(French's) *Gravy Makins*	½ cup	50
*Dietetic (Weight Watchers):		
Brown	½ cup	16
Brown, with mushroom	½ cup	24
Brown, with onion	½ cup	26
Chicken	½ cup	20
GRAVY WITH MEAT OR TURKEY,		
Frozen:		
(Banquet):		
Entree for One, & sliced beef	4 oz.	90
Family Entree, & sliced turkey	32-oz. pkg.	640
(Morton) Light, sliced turkey	8 oz.	270
(Swanson) sliced beef	8-oz. entree	200
GREAT BEGINNINGS		
(Hormel):		
With chunky beef	5 oz.	136
With chunky chicken	5 oz.	147
With chunky turkey	5 oz.	138
GREENS, MIXED, canned:		
(Allens)	½ cup	25
(Sunshine) solids & liq.	½ cup	20
GRENADINE (Garnier) no alcohol	1 fl. oz	103
GUAVA	1 guava	48
GUAVA NECTAR (Libby's)	6 fl. oz.	70

H

Food and Description	Measure or Quantity	Calories
HADDOCK:		
Fried, breaded	4″ × 3″ × ½″ fillet	165
Frozen:		
(Gorton's) *Light Recipe,* fillet entree	1 piece	260
(Mrs. Paul's) breaded & fried crispy, crunchy	2-oz. fillet	140
(Van de Kamp's) batter dipped, french fried	2-oz. piece	120
(Weight Watchers) with stuffing, 2-compartment	7-oz. pkg.	205
Smoked	4-oz. serving	117
HALIBUT:		
Broiled	4″ × 3″ × ½″ steak	214
Frozen (Van de Kamp's) batter dipped, french fried	½ of 8-oz. pkg.	260
HAM:		
Canned:		
(Hormel):		
Black Label (3- or 5-lb. size)	4 oz.	140
Chunk	6¾-oz. serving	310
Patties	1 patty	180
(Oscar Mayer) *Jubilee,* extra lean, cooked	1-oz. serving	31
(Swift) *Premium*	1¾-oz. slice	111
Deviled:		
(Hormel)	1 T.	35
(Libby's)	1 T.	43
(Underwood)	1 T.	49
Packaged:		
(Carl Buddig) smoked	1 oz.	50
(Eckrich):		
Loaf	1 oz.	70
Cooked or imported, Danish	1.2-oz. slice	30
(Hormel):		
Black, or red peppered or frozen	1 slice	25
Chopped	1 slice	55

81

Food and Description	Measure or Quantity	Calories
(Oscar Mayer):		
Chopped	1-oz. slice	64
Cooked, smoked	1-oz. slice	34
Jubilee, boneless:		
Sliced	8-oz. slice	232
Steak, 95% fat free	2-oz. steak	59
HAM & CHEESE:		
(Eckrich) loaf	1-oz. serving	60
(Hormel) loaf	1-oz. serving	65
HAM DINNER, frozen:		
(Banquet) American Favorites	10-oz. dinner	532
(Morton)	10-oz. dinner	301
HAM SALAD, canned (Carnation)	¼ of 7½-oz. can	110
HAM SALAD SPREAD		
(Oscar Mayer)	1 oz.	62
HAMBURGER (See *McDONALD'S, BURGER KING, DAIRY QUEEN, WHITE CASTLE,* etc.)		
HAMBURGER MIX:		
Hamburger Helper		
(General Mills):		
Beef noodle, tomato or pizza dish	⅕ pkg.	320
Cheeseburger Macaroni	⅕ pkg.	360
Hash	⅕ pkg.	300
Lasagna	⅕ pkg.	330
Potatoes au gratin	⅕ pkg.	320
Stew	⅕ pkg.	290
Make a Better Burger (Lipton)		
mildly seasoned or onion	⅕ pkg.	30
HAMBURGER SEASONING MIX:		
*(Durkee)	1 cup	663
(French's)	1-oz. pkg.	100
HARDEE'S:		
Chef's salad	1 serving	310
Garden salad	1 serving	245
Seafood salad	1 serving	170
Side salad	1 serving	90
Bacon bits	1 packet	15
Crackers	1 packet	35
Croutons	1 packet	30
Blue cheese dressing	1 packet	210
Lo-cal French dressing	1 packet	140
House dressing	1 packet	290
Lo-cal Italian dressing	1 packet	90
Thousand Island dressing	1 packet	250
HAWAIIAN PUNCH:		
Canned regular:		
Cherry or grape	6 fl. oz.	90
Orange	6 fl. oz.	100

Food and Description	Measure or Quantity	Calories
Canned, dietetic, punch	6 fl. oz.	30
HEADCHEESE (Oscar Mayer)	1-oz. serving	55
HERRING, canned (Vita):		
Cocktail, drained	8-oz. jar	342
In cream sauce	8-oz. jar	397
Tastee Bits, drained	8-oz. jar	361
HERRING, SMOKED, kippered	4-oz. serving	239
HICKORY NUT, shelled	1 oz.	191
HO-HO (Hostess)	1-oz. piece	120
HOMINY, canned (Allens)		
golden, solids & liq.	½ cup	80
HOMINY GRITS:		
Dry:		
(Albers)	1½ oz.	150
(Aunt Jemima)	3 T.	102
(Quaker):		
Regular	3 T.	101
Instant:		
Regular	.8-oz. packet	79
With imitation bacon or ham	1-oz. packet	101
Cooked	1 cup	125
HONEY, strained	1 T.	61
HONEYCOMB, cereal (Post) regular	1⅓ cups	112
HONEYDEW	2" × 7" wedge	31
HONEY SMACKS, cereal (Kellogg's)	¾ cup	110
HORSERADISH:		
Raw, pared	1 oz.	25
Prepared (Gold's)	1 tsp.	3
HOSTESS O'S (Hostess)	2¾-oz. piece	277

I

Food and Description	Measure or Quantity	Calories
ICE CREAM (Listed by type, such as sandwich, or *Whammy*, or by flavor—see also FROZEN DESSERT):		
Almond amaretto (Baskin-Robbins)	4 fl. oz.	280
Bar:		
(Good Humor) vanilla, chocolate coated	3-fl.-oz. piece	170
(Häagen-Dazs):		
Chocolate, dark chocolate coating	1 piece	360
Vanilla, milk chocolate coated	1 bar	330
Bon Bon (Carnation) vanilla	1 piece	33
Brandied black cherry (Häagen-Dazs)	4 fl. oz.	220
Butter Almond (Breyers)	½ cup	170
Butter pecan:		
(Breyer's)	¼ pt.	180
(Good Humor) bulk	4 fl. oz.	150
(Häagen-Dazs)	4 fl. oz.	312
Cappuccino:		
(Baskin-Robbins) chip	4 fl. oz.	310
(Häagen-Dazs)	4 fl. oz.	252
Chocolate:		
(Baskin-Robbins):		
Regular	4 fl. oz.	264
Mousse Royale	4 fl. oz.	293
(Breyers)	½ cup	160
(Good Humor) bulk	4 fl. oz.	130
(Häagen-Dazs) mint	4 fl. oz.	300
(Howard Johnson's)	½ cup	221
Chocolate chip (Häagen-Dazs)	4 fl. oz.	280
Chocolate chip cookie (Good Humor) vanilla	1 sandwich	246
Chocolate eclair (Good Humor) bar	3-fl.-oz piece	187
Chocolate malt bar (Good Humor)	3-fl. oz. bar	186
Chocolate raspberry truffle (Baskin-Robbins)	4 fl. oz.	310
Coffee:		
(Breyers)	½ cup	140

84

Food and Description	Measure or Quantity	Calories
(Häagen-Dazs) chip	4 fl. oz.	272
Cookies & cream:		
(Breyer's)	½ cup	170
(Häagen-Dazs)	4 fl. oz.	272
(Sealtest)	½ cup	150
Cookie sandwich (Good Humor)	2.7 fl. oz. piece	290
Eskimo Pie, vanilla with chocolate coating	3-fl.-oz. bar	180
Eskimo, Thin Mint, with chocolate coating	2-fl.-oz. bar	140
Fat Frog (Good Humor)	3-fl.-oz. pop	154
Fudge royal (Sealtest)	½ cup	140
Grand marnier (Baskin-Robbins)	4 fl. oz.	240
Heart (Good Humor)	4-fl.-oz. pop	200
Honey (Häagen-Dazs)	4 fl. oz.	256
Jamocha (Baskin-Robbins)	1 scoop (2½ fl. oz.)	146
Key lime & cream (Häagen-Dazs)	4 fl. oz.	192
Macadamia nut (Häagen-Dazs)	4 fl. oz.	320
Maple walnut (Häagen-Dazs)	4 fl. oz.	312
Mint chocolate chip (Breyers)	½ cup	170
Oreo, Cookies 'n Cream:		
Bulk	3 fl. oz.	140
Sandwich	1 piece	240
Peach (Häagen-Dazs)	4 fl. oz.	212
Pralines 'N Cream (Baskin-Robbins)	1 scoop (2½ fl. oz.)	177
Rocky Road (Baskin-Robbins)	4 fl. oz.	291
Rum raisin (Häagen-Dazs)	4 fl. oz.	240
Sandwich (Good Humor) vanilla	2½-oz. piece	161
Shark Bar (Good Humor)	3-fl.-oz. pop	63
Strawberry:		
(Baskin-Robbins) wild, light	4 fl. oz.	90
(Breyers)	½ cup	130
(Häagen-Dazs)	4 fl. oz.	232
(Howard Johnson's)	½ cup	187
Toasted almond bar (Good Humor)	3-fl.-oz. piece	193
Vanilla:		
(Baskin-Robbins) regular	4 fl. oz.	235
(Häagen-Dazs)	4 fl. oz.	250
(Howard Johnson's)	½ cup	210
(Meadow Gold)	½ cup	140
(Sealtest)	½ cup	140
Vanilla slice (Good Humor):		
Regular	3.2-fl.-oz. slice	110
Calorie controlled	3.2-fl.-oz. slice	60
Vanilla swiss almond (Häagen-Dazs)	4 fl. oz.	300
Whammy (Good Humor) assorted	1.6-oz. piece	95

Food and Description	Measure or Quantity	Calories
ICE CREAM CONE, cone only		
(Comet) regular	1 piece	40
ICE CREAM CUP, cup only		
(Comet) regular	1 cup	20
*ICE CREAM MIX (Salada)		
any flavor	1 cup	310
ICE MILK:		
Hardened	¼ pt.	100
Soft-serve	¼ pt.	133
(Dean) *Count Calorie*	¼ pt.	99
(Light 'n Lively) coffee	½ cup	100
(Meadow Gold) vanilla, 4% fat	¼ pt.	95
ITALIAN DINNER, frozen		
(Banquet)	12-oz. dinner	597

J

Food and Description	Measure or Quantity	Calories
JACK IN THE BOX RESTAURANT:		
Breakfast Jack	4.4-oz. serving	307
Burger:		
Regular	3.4-oz. serving	267
Cheeseburger:		
Regular	4-oz. serving	315
Bacon	8.1-oz. serving	705
Ultimate	9.9-oz. serving	942
Ham & Swiss	9.1-oz. serving	754
Jumbo Jack:		
Regular	7.8-oz. serving	584
With cheese	8.5-oz. serving	677
Monterey Burger	9.9-oz. serving	865
Mushroom	6.4-oz. serving	470
Swiss & bacon	6.6-oz. serving	678
Canadian crescent	4.7-oz. serving	452
Cheesecake	3.5-oz. serving	309
Chicken strips	1 piece	87
Chicken supreme sandwich	8.1-oz. serving	575
Club pita sandwich, excluding sauce	6.3-oz. serving	277
Coffee, black	8 fl. oz.	2
Egg, scrambled, platter	8.8-oz. serving	662
Egg roll	1 piece	135
Fish supreme sandwich	8-oz. sandwich	554
French fries:		
Regular	2.4-oz. order	221
Large	3.8-oz. order	353
Jumbo	4.8-oz. order	442
Jelly, grape	.5-oz. serving	38
Ketchup	1 serving	10
Mayonnaise	1 serving	152
Milk, low fat	8 fl. oz.	122
Milk shake:		
Chocolate	11.4-oz. serving	320
Strawberry	11.4-oz. serving	320
Vanilla	11.2-oz. serving	320
Mustard	1 serving	8
Nachos:		
Cheese	6-oz. serving	571

Food and Description	Measure or Quantity	Calories
Supreme	11.9-oz. serving	787
Onion rings	3.8-oz. serving	382
Orange juice	6.5-oz. serving	80
Pancake platter	8.1-oz. serving	612
Salad:		
Chef	13-oz. salad	295
Mexican chicken	15.2-oz. salad	443
Side	3.9-oz. salad	51
Taco	12.6-oz. salad	377
Salad dressing:		
Regular:		
Blue cheese	1.2-oz. serving	131
Buttermilk	1.2-oz. serving	181
Thousand Island	1.2-oz. serving	156
Dietetic or low calorie, French	1.2-oz. serving	80
Sauce:		
A-1	1.8-oz. serving	35
BBQ	.9-oz. serving	44
Guacamole	.9-oz. serving	55
Mayo-mustard	.8-oz. serving	124
Mayo-onion	.8-oz. serving	143
Salsa	.9-oz. serving	8
Seafood cocktail	1-oz. serving	32
Sweet & sour	1-oz. serving	40
Sausage crescent	5.5-oz. serving	585
Shrimp	1 piece (.3 oz.)	27
Soft drink:		
Sweetened:		
Coca-Cola Classic	12 fl. oz.	144
Dr. Pepper	12 fl. oz.	144
Root beer, *Ramblin'*	12 fl. oz.	176
Sprite	12 fl. oz.	144
Diet, *Coca-Cola*	12 fl. oz.	Tr.
Supreme crescent	5.1-oz. serving	547
Syrup, pancake	1.5-oz. serving	121
Taco:		
Regular	2.9-oz. serving	191
Super	4.8-oz. serving	288
Tea, iced, plain	12 fl. oz.	3
Turnover, hot apple	4.2-oz. piece	410
JELL-O FRUIT BAR	1 bar	45
JELL-O FRUIT & CREAM BAR	1 bar	72
JELL-O GELATIN POPS	1 pop	35
JELL-O PUDDING POPS:		
Chocolate, chocolate with chocolate chips & vanilla with chocolate chips	1 bar	80
Chocolate covered chocolate & vanilla	1 bar	130

Food and Description	Measure or Quantity	Calories
JELLY, sweetened (See also individual flavors)		
(Crosse & Blackwell) all flavors	1 T.	51
JERUSALEM ARTICHOKE, pared	4 oz.	75
JOHANNISBERG RIESLING WINE		
(Louis M. Martini)	3 fl. oz.	68

K

Food and Description	Measure or Quantity	Calories
KABOOM, cereal (General Mills)	1 cup	110
KALE:		
Boiled, leaves only	4 oz.	110
Canned (Allen's) chopped, solids & liq.	½ cup	25
Frozen:		
(Birds Eye) chopped	⅓ pkg.	32
(McKenzie) chopped	3⅓ oz.	30
(Southland) chopped	⅕ of 16-oz. pkg.	25
KARO SYRUP (See SYRUP)		
KEFIR (Alta-Dena Dairy):		
Plain	1 cup	180
Flavored	1 cup	190
KIDNEY:		
Beef, braised	4 oz.	286
Calf, raw	4 oz.	128
Lamb, raw	4 oz.	119
KIELBASA (see **SAUSAGE**, Polish-style)		
KING VITAMAN, cereal (Quaker)	1¼ cups	113
KIPPER SNACKS (King David Brand) Norwegian	3¼-oz. can	195
KIX, cereal	1½ cups	110
KNOCKWURST	1 oz.	79
***KOOL-AID** (General Foods):		
Unsweetened (sugar to be added)	8 fl. oz.	98
Pre-sweetened:		
Regular, sugar sweetened:		
Apple or sunshine punch	8 fl. oz.	96
Cherry or grape	8 fl. oz.	89
Tropical punch	8 fl. oz.	99
Dietetic, sugar-free:		
Cherry or grape	8 fl. oz.	2
Sunshine punch	8 fl. oz.	4
KUMQUAT, flesh & skin	5 oz.	74

L

Food and Description	Measure or Quantity	Calories
LAMB:		
Leg:		
Roasted, lean & fat	3 oz.	237
Roasted, lean only	3 oz.	158

Loin, one 5-oz. chop (weighed with
  bone before cooking)
  will give you:		

Lean & fat	2.8 oz.	280
Lean only	2.3 oz.	122

Rib, one 5-oz. chop (weighed with
  bone before cooking)
  will give you:		

Lean & fat	2.9 oz.	334
Lean only	2 oz.	118
Shoulder:		
Roasted, lean & fat	3 oz.	287
Roasted, lean only	3 oz.	174
LASAGNA:		
Canned (Hormel) *Short Orders*	7½-oz. can	260
Frozen:		
(Armour) *Dinner Classics*	10-oz. meal	380
(Buitoni):		
Regular	9-oz. serving	342
Al forno	8-oz. serving	327
Meat sauce	5-oz. serving	212
(Celentano):		
Regular	½ of 16-oz. pkg.	320
Primavera	11-oz. pkg.	300
(Conagra) *Light & Elegant*	11¼-oz. entree	280
(Le Menu) vegetable	11-oz. dinner	360
(Stouffer's) *Lean Cuisine*	11-oz. meal	240
(Swanson):		
Hungry Man, with meat	18¾-oz. dinner	730
Main Course, with meat	13¼-oz. entree	450
(Weight Watcher's) regular	12-oz. meal	360
LEEKS	4 oz.	59
LEMON:		
Whole	2⅛" lemon	22
Peeled	2⅛" lemon	20

Food and Description	Measure or Quantity	Calories
LEMONADE:		
Canned:		
Capri Sun	6¾ fl. oz.	63
Country Time	6 fl. oz.	69
Chilled (Minute Maid) regular or pink	6 fl. oz.	79
*Frozen:		
Country Time, regular or pink	6 fl. oz.	68
Minute Maid	6 fl. oz.	74
*Mix:		
Regular:		
Country Time, regular or pink	6 fl. oz.	68
(Hi-C)	6 fl. oz.	76
Kool-Aid, sweetened, regular or pink	6 fl. oz.	65
Lemon Tree (Lipton)	6 fl. oz.	68
Dietetic:		
Crystal Light	8 fl. oz.	4
Kool-Aid	6 fl. oz.	3
(Sunkist)	8 fl. oz.	8
LEMONADE BAR (Sunkist)	3-fl.-oz. bar	70
LEMON EXTRACT (Virginia Dare)	1 tsp.	21
LEMON JUICE:		
Canned, *ReaLemon*	1 T.	3
*Frozen (Minute Maid) unsweetened	1 fl. oz.	77
*LEMON-LIMEADE DRINK, *Crystal-Light*	8 fl. oz.	4
LEMON PEEL, candied	1 oz.	90
LENTIL, cooked, drained	½ cup	107
LETTUCE:		
Bibb or Boston	4″ head	23
Cos or Romaine, shredded or broken into pieces	½ cup	4
Grand Rapids, Salad Bowl or Simpson	2 large leaves	9
Iceberg, New York or Great Lakes	¼ of 4¾″ head	15
LIFE, cereal (Quaker) regular or cinnamon	⅔ cup	105
LIL' ANGELS (Hostess)	1-oz. piece	90
LIME, peeled	2″ dia.	15
*LIMEADE, frozen (Minute Maid)	6 fl. oz.	75
LIME JUICE, *ReaLime*	1 T.	2
LINGUINI, frozen (Stouffer's) clam sauce	10½ oz.	285
LIVER:		
Beef:		
Fried	6½″ × 2⅜″ × ⅜″ slice	195
Cooked (Swift)	3.2-oz. serving	141
Calf, fried	6½″ × 2⅛″ × ⅜″ slice	222

Food and Description	Measure or Quantity	Calories
Chicken, simmered	2″ × 2″ × ⅝″ piece	41
LIVERWURST SPREAD (Hormel)	1-oz. serving	70
LOBSTER:		
Cooked, meat only	1 cup	138
Canned, meat only	4-oz. serving	108
Frozen, South African lobster tail		
3 in 8-oz. pkg.	1 piece	87
4 in 8-oz. pkg.	1 piece	65
5 in 8-oz. pkg.	1 piece	51
LOBSTER NEWBURG	1 cup	485
LOBSTER PASTE, canned	1-oz. serving	51
LOBSTER SALAD	4-oz. serving	125
LONG ISLAND TEA COCKTAIL		
(Mr. Boston) 12½% alcohol	3 fl. oz.	93
LONG JOHN SILVER'S:		
Catfish fillet	2.7-oz. piece	203
Catsup	.4 oz.	12
Chicken plank	1.4-oz. piece	104
Chicken sandwich	6.1-oz. sandwich	562
Chowder, clam	1 order	128
Clams, breaded	4.7-oz. order	526
Coleslaw	3½ oz. (drained on fork)	182
Corn on the cob	5.3-oz. ear	176
Cracker	1 piece	12
Drinks:		
Regular, carbonated or non-carbonated	10 fl. oz.	120
Dietetic	10 fl. oz.	Tr.
Fish fillet:		
Baked, with sauce	5.5-oz. serving	151
Batter fried	3-oz. piece	202
Kitchen breaded	2-oz. piece	122
Fish sandwich	6.4-oz. sandwich	555
Fryer	3-oz. serving	247
Hush puppies	.85-oz. piece	72
Oyster, breaded, fried	.7-oz. piece	60
Peg Leg, battered	1-oz. piece	91
Pie:		
Apple	4-oz. piece	280
Cherry	4-oz. piece	294
Lemon meringue	3½-oz. piece	200
Pecan	4-oz. piece	446
Pumpkin	4-oz. piece	251
Scallop, batter fried	.7-oz. piece	53
Seafood salad	5.8 oz. serving	386
Seafood sauce	1.2-oz. serving	34
Shrimp:		
Batter fried	.6-oz. piece	47

Food and Description	Measure or Quantity	Calories
Breaded, fried	4.7-oz. order	388
Chilled	.2-oz. piece	6
Tartar sauce	1-oz. serving	119
Vegetables, mixed	4-oz. serving	54
LOQUAT, fresh, flesh only	2 oz.	27
LUCKY CHARMS, cereal (General Mills)	1 cup	110
LUNCHEON MEAT (See also individual listings such as BOLOGNA, HAM, etc.):		
Banquet loaf (Eckrich)	¾-oz. slice	50
Bar-B-Que loaf (Oscar Mayer) 90% fat free	1-oz. slice	48
Beef, jellied loaf (Hormel)	1.2-oz. slice	45
Gourmet loaf (Eckrich)	1-oz. slice	35
Ham & cheese (See HAM & CHEESE)		
Ham roll sausage (Oscar Mayer)	1-oz. slice	43
Honey loaf:		
(Eckrich)	1-oz. slice	40
(Hormel)	1 slice	55
(Oscar Mayer)	1-oz. slice	35
Iowa brand (Hormel)	1 slice	45
Liver cheese (Oscar Mayer)	1.3-oz. slice	116
Liver loaf (Hormel)	1 slice	80
Macaroni-cheese loaf (Eckrich)	1-oz. slice	68
Meat loaf	1-oz. serving	57
New England brand sliced sausage:		
(Eckrich)	1-oz. slice	35
(Oscar Mayer) 92% fat free	.8-oz. slice	22
Old fashioned loaf (Oscar Mayer)	1-oz. slice	64
Olive loaf:		
(Eckrich)	1-oz. slice	80
(Hormel)	1-oz. slice	55
(Oscar Mayer)	1-oz. slice	62
Peppered loaf:		
(Eckrich)	1-oz. slice	40
(Hormel) Light & Lean	1 slice	50
(Oscar Mayer) 93% fat free	1-oz. slice	43
Pickle loaf:		
(Eckrich)	1-oz. slice	80
(Hormel)	1 slice	60
Pickle & pimiento (Oscar Mayer)	1-oz. slice	63
Pressed luncheon sausage (Oscar Mayer)	.8-oz. slice	35
Spiced (Hormel)	1 slice	75

M

Food and Description	Measure or Quantity	Calories
MACADAMIA NUT		
(Royal Hawaiian)	1 oz.	197
MACARONI:		
Cooked:		
8-10 minutes, firm	1 cup	192
14-20 minutes, tender	1 cup	155
Canned (Franco-American) *PizzOs*	7½-oz. can	170
Frozen:		
(Morton) & beef	10-oz. dinner	245
(Swanson) & beef	12-oz. dinner	360
MACARONI & CHEESE:		
Canned:		
(Franco-American) regular		
or elbow	7⅜-oz. serving	170
(Hormel) *Short Orders*	7½-oz. can	170
Frozen:		
(Banquet):		
Casserole	8-oz. pkg.	344
Dinner	9-oz. dinner	334
(Celentano) baked	½ of 12-oz. pkg.	290
(Conagra) *Light & Elegant*	9-oz. entree	300
(Morton)	20-oz. casserole	648
(Stouffer's)	6-oz. serving	260
(Swanson)	12¼-oz. dinner	380
Mix:		
(Golden Grain) deluxe	¼ pkg.	190
*(Kraft):		
Regular, plain	¼ box	190
Velveeta, shells	¼ box	270
*(Prince)	¾ cup	268
MACARONI & CHEESE PIE,		
frozen (Swanson)	7-oz. pie	210
MACARONI SALAD, canned		
(Nalley's)	4-oz. serving	206
MACKEREL, Atlantic, broiled with fat	8½" × 2½" × ½" fillet	248
MAGIC SHELL (Smucker's)	1 T.	95
MAI TAI COCKTAIL MIX (Holland House):		
Instant	.56-oz. envelope	64

Food and Description	Measure or Quantity	Calories
Liquid	1 oz.	32
MALTED MILK MIX (Carnation):		
Chocolate	3 heaping tsps.	85
Natural	3 heaping tsps.	88
MALT LIQUOR, *Colt 45*	12 fl. oz.	156
MALT-O-MEAL, cereal	1 T.	33
MANDARIN ORANGE (See TANGERINE)		
MANGO, fresh	1 med. mango	88
MANGO NECTAR (Libby's)	6 fl. oz.	60
MANHATTAN COCKTAIL (Mr. Boston) 20% alcohol	3 fl. oz.	123
MANHATTAN COCKTAIL MIX (Holland House) liquid	1 oz.	28
MANICOTTI, frozen:		
(Buitoni):		
Cheese	5.5 oz.	310
Florentine	2 manicotti	284
(Celentano):		
Without sauce	1 manicotti	85
With sauce	1 manicotti	150
MANWICH (Hunt's)	5.8-oz. serving	310
MAPLE SYRUP (See SYRUP, Maple)		
MARGARINE:		
Regular:	1 pat (1″ × 1.3″ × 1″, 5 grams)	36
(Mazola)	1 T.	104
(Parkay) regular, soft or squeeze	1 T.	101
Imitation or dietetic:		
(Parkay)	1 T.	55
(Weight Watchers)	1 T.	50
Whipped (Blue Bonnet; Miracle; Parkay)	1 T.	67
MARGARITA COCKTAIL (Mr. Boston):		
Regular	3 fl. oz.	105
Strawberry	3 fl. oz.	138
MARINADE MIX:		
Chicken (Adolph's)	1-oz. packet	64
Meat:		
(French's)	1-oz. pkg.	80
(Kikkoman)	1-oz. pkg.	64
MARJORAM (French's)	1 tsp.	4
MARMALADE:		
Sweetened:		
(Home Brands)	1 T.	52
(Keiller)	1 T.	60

Food and Description	Measure or Quantity	Calories
(Smucker's)	1 T.	53
Dietetic:		
(Estee; Louis Sherry)	1 T.	6
(Featherweight)	1 T.	16
(S&W) *Nutradiet*, red label	1 T.	12
MARSHMALLOW FLUFF	1 heaping tsp.	59
MARSHMALLOW KRISPIES, cereal		
(Kellogg's)	1¼ cups	140
MARTINI COCKTAIL (Mr. Boston):		
Gin, extra dry, 20% alcohol	3 fl. oz.	99
Vodka, 20% alcohol	3 fl. oz.	102
MASA HARINA (Quaker)	⅓ cup	137
MASA TRIGO (Quaker)	⅓ cup	149
MATZO (Manischewitz):		
Regular:		
Plain	1-oz piece	110
Egg	1 cracker	108
Miniature	1 cracker	9
Tam Tam	1 cracker	15
Wheat	1 cracker	9
Dietetic:		
Tam Tam, unsalted	1 cracker	14
Thins	.8 oz. piece	91
MATZO FARFEL		
(Manischewitz)	½ cup	143
MAYONNAISE:		
Real:		
Hellmann's (Best Foods)	1 T.	103
(Kraft)	1 T.	100
(Rokeach)	1 T.	100
Imitation or dietetic:		
(Estee)	1 T.	100
(Diet Delight) *Mayo-Lite*	1 T.	24
(Featherweight) *Soyamaise*	1 T.	100
(Kraft) light	1 T.	45
(Pritikin) *Sweetlite*	1 T.	50
(Weight Watchers)	1 T.	40
MAYPO, cereal:		
30-second	¼ cup	89
Vermont style	¼ cup	121
McDONALD'S:		
Big Mac	1 hamburger	570
Biscuit:		
Plain	1 order	330
With bacon, egg & cheese	1 order	483
With sausage	1 order	467
With sausage & egg	1 order	585
Cheeseburger	1 cheeseburger	318
Chicken McNuggets	1 serving	323

Food and Description	Measure or Quantity	Calories
Chicken McNuggets Sauce:		
Barbecue	1.1-oz. serving	60
Honey	.5-oz. serving	50
Hot mustard or sweet & sour	1.1-oz. serving	63
Cookies:		
Chocolate chip	1 package	342
McDonaldland	1 package	308
Egg McMuffin	1 serving	340
Egg, scrambled	1 serving	180
English muffin, with butter	1 muffin	186
Filet-O-Fish	1 sandwich	435
Grapefruit juice	6 fl. oz.	75
Hamburger	1 hamburger	263
Hot cakes with butter & syrup	1 serving	500
Pie:		
Apple	1 pie	253
Cherry	1 pie	260
Potato:		
Fried	1 regular order	220
Hash browns	1 order	125
Quarter Pounder:		
Regular	1 hamburger	427
With cheese	1 hamburger	525
Salad:		
Chef's salad	*1 serving*	*230*
Garden salad	*1 serving*	*110*
Chicken oriental salad	*1 serving*	*140*
Shrimp salad	*1 serving*	*105*
Side salad	*1 serving*	*55*
Salad Bar:		
Bacon bits	*1 packet*	*15*
Chow mein noodles	*1 packet*	*45*
Croutons	*1 packet*	*50*
Salad Dressings:		
Blue cheese	1 packet	345
French	1 packet	230
House	1 packet	330
Oriental	1 packet	95
Thousand Island	1 packet	390
Lo-cal vinaigrette	1 packet	60
Sausage McMuffin:		
Plain	1 sandwich	427
With egg	1 sandwich	517
Sausage, pork	1 serving	210
Shake:		
Chocolate	1 serving	383
Strawberry	1 serving	362
Vanilla	1 serving	352
Sundae:		

Food and Description	Measure or Quantity	Calories
Caramel	1 serving	361
Hot fudge	1 serving	357
Strawberry	1 serving	320
MEATBALL DINNER or ENTREE, frozen:		
(Green Giant) sweet & sour	9.9-oz. entree	370
(Swanson)	8¼-oz. entree	290
***MEATBALL SEASONING MIX**		
(Durkee) *Italian style*	1 cup	619
MEATBALL STEW:		
Canned *Dinty Moore* (Hormel)	7½-oz. serving	245
Frozen (Stouffer's) *Lean Cuisine*	10-oz. serving	240
MEATBALLS, SWEDISH, frozen:		
(Armour) *Dinner Classics*	11½-oz. meal	470
(Stouffer's) with noodles	11-oz. pkg.	475
MEAT LOAF DINNER, frozen:		
(Banquet):		
Dinner	11-oz. dinner	395
Entree for One	5-oz.	240
(Morton)	11-oz. dinner	371
(Swanson) with tomato sauce	9-oz. entree	310
MEAT LOAF SEASONING MIX:		
*(Bell's)	4½ oz.	300
(Contadina)	3¾-oz. pkg.	360
MEAT, POTTED:		
(Hormel)	1 T.	30
(Libby's)	1-oz. serving	55
MEAT TENDERIZER:		
Regular (Adolph's; McCormick)	1 tsp.	2
Seasoned (McCormick)	1 tsp.	5
MELBA TOAST, salted (Old London):		
Garlic, onion or white rounds	1 piece	10
Pumpernickel, rye, wheat or white	1 piece	17
MELON BALL, in syrup, frozen	½ cup	72
MENUDO, canned (Hormel) *Casa Grande*	7½-oz. can	90
MERLOT WINE (Louis M. Martini) 12½% alcohol	3 fl. oz.	63
MEXICALI DOGS, frozen (Hormel)	5-oz. serving	400
MEXICAN DINNER, frozen:		
(Morton)	11-oz. dinner	300
(Swanson)	16-oz. dinner	580
(Van de Kamp's) combination	11½-oz. dinner	420
***MILK BREAK BARS** (Pillsbury):		
Chocolate or chocolate mint	1 bar	230
Natural	1 bar	220
MILK, CONDENSED, *Eagle Brand* (Borden)	1 T.	64

Food and Description	Measure or Quantity	Calories
*MILK, DRY, non-fat, instant (Alba; Carnation; Pet; *Sanalac*)	1 cup	80
MILK, EVAPORATED:		
Regular:		
(Carnation)	1 fl. oz.	42
(Pet)	1 fl. oz.	43
Filled (Pet)	½ cup	150
Low fat (Carnation)	1 fl. oz.	27
Skimmed, (Carnation; *Pet 99*)	1 fl. oz.	25
MILK, FRESH:		
Buttermilk (Friendship)	8 fl. oz.	120
Chocolate:		
(Borden) *Dutch Brand*	8 fl. oz.	180
(Hershey's)	8 fl. oz.	190
(Johanna):		
Regular	8 fl. oz.	200
Lowfat	8 fl. oz.	150
(Nestlé) *Quik*	8 fl. oz.	220
Low fat:		
(Borden):		
1% milkfat	8 fl. oz.	100
2% milkfat, *Hi-Protein Brand*	8 fl. oz.	140
(Johanna):		
Regular:		
1% lowfat	8 fl. oz.	100
2% lowfat, regular	8 fl. oz.	120
Buttermilk	8 fl. oz.	120
Skim (Dairylea; Meadow Gold)	1 cup	90
Whole:		
(Borden) regular or high calcium	8 fl. oz.	150
(Johanna)	8 fl. oz.	150
MILK, GOAT, whole	1 cup	163
MILK, HUMAN	1 cup	163
MILK MAKERS (Swiss Miss):		
Chocolate, malted or strawberry	1 envelope or 1 tsp.	18
*Chocolate, malted or strawberry	8 fl. oz.	100
MILNOT, dairy vegetable blend	1 fl. oz.	38
MINERAL WATER (La Croix)	Any quantity	0
MINI-WHEATS, cereal (Kellogg's) frosted	1 biscuit	28
MINT LEAVES	½ oz.	4
MOLASSES:		
Barbados	1 T.	51
Blackstrap	1 T.	40
Dark (Brer Rabbit)	1 T.	33
Light	1 T.	48
Medium	1 T.	44
Unsulphured (Grandma's)	1 T.	60
MORTADELLA sausage	1 oz.	89

Food and Description	Measure or Quantity	Calories
MOST, cereal (Kellogg's)	½ cup	100
MOUSSE:		
Canned, dietetic (Featherweight) chocolate	½ cup	100
*Mix, dietetic (Pritikin):		
Chocolate	½ cup	80
Lemon or strawberry	½ cup	70
MUFFIN:		
Apple (Pepperidge Farm) with spice	1 muffin	170
Blueberry:		
(Morton) rounds	1.5-oz. muffin	110
(Pepperidge Farm)	1.9-oz. muffin	180
Bran (Pepperidge Farm)	1 muffin	180
Carrot walnut (Pepperidge Farm)	1 muffin	170
Chocolate chip (Pepperidge Farm)	1 muffin	170
Corn:		
(Morton)	1.7-oz. muffin	130
(Pepperidge Farm)	1.9-oz. muffin	180
English:		
(Pepperidge Farm):		
Plain	2-oz. muffin	140
Cinnamon, raisin	2-oz. muffin	150
Roman Meal	2.3-oz. muffin	150
(Thomas'):		
Regular or frozen or sourdough	2-oz. muffin	133
Raisin	2.2-oz. muffin	153
(Wonder)	2-oz. muffin	130
Plain	1.4-oz. muffin	118
Sourdough (Wonder)	2-oz. muffin	130
MUFFIN MIX:		
Blueberry:		
*(Betty Crocker) wild	1 muffin	120
(Duncan Hines)	1/12 pkg.	99
Bran:		
(Duncan Hines)	1/12 pkg.	97
(Elam's) natural	1 T.	23
*Cherry (Betty Crocker)	1/12 pkg.	120
Corn:		
*(Betty Crocker)	1 muffin	160
*(Dromedary)	1 muffin	120
MULLIGAN STEW, canned, *Dinty Moore, Short Orders* (Hormel)	7½-oz. can	230
MUSCATEL WINE (Gallo)		
14% alcohol	3 fl. oz.	86
MUSHROOM:		
Raw, whole	½ lb.	62
Raw, trimmed, sliced	½ cup	10
Canned (Green Giant) solids & liq., whole or sliced:		

Food and Description	Measure or Quantity	Calories
Regular	2-oz. serving	14
B & B	1½-oz. serving	18
Frozen (Larsen)	3½ oz.	30
MUSHROOM, CHINESE, dried	1 oz.	81
MUSSEL, in shell	1 lb.	153
MUSTARD:		
Powder (French's)	1 tsp.	9
Prepared:		
Brown (French's; Gulden's)	1 tsp.	5
Chinese (Chun King)	1 tsp.	5
Dijon, *Grey Poupon*	1 tsp.	6
Horseradish (Nalley's)	1 tsp.	5
Yellow (Gulden's)	1 tsp.	5
MUSTARD GREENS:		
Canned (Allens) solids & liq.	½ cup	20
Frozen:		
(Birds Eye)	⅓ pkg.	25
(Frosty Acres)	3.3 oz.	20
(Southland)	⅓ of 16-oz. pkg.	20
MUSTARD SPINACH:		
Raw	1 lb.	100
Boiled, drained, no added salt	4-oz. serving	18

N

Food and Description	Measure or Quantity	Calories
NATHAN'S:		
French fries	Regular order	550
Hamburger	1 sandwich	360
Hot dog & roll	1 order	290
NATURAL CEREAL:		
Familia:		
Regular	½ cup	187
Bran	½ cup	166
No added sugar	½ cup	181
Heartland:		
Plain, coconut or raisin	¼ cup	130
Trail mix	¼ cup	120
(Quaker):		
Hot, whole wheat	⅓ cup	106
100%	¼ cup	138
100% with raisins & dates	¼ cup	134
NATURE SNACKS (Sun-Maid):		
Carob Crunch	1 oz.	143
Carob Peanut	1¼ oz.	190
Carob Raisin or Yogurt Raisin	1¼ oz.	160
Tahitian Treat or Yogurt Crunch	1 oz.	123
NECTARINE, flesh only	4 oz.	73
NOODLE:		
Cooked, 1½″ strips	1 cup	200
Dry (Pennsylvania Dutch Brand) broad	1 oz.	105
NOODLE, CHOW MEIN:		
(Chun King)	1 oz.	139
(La Choy)	½ cup (1 oz.)	150
NOODLE MIX:		
*(Betty Crocker):		
Fettucini Alfredo	¼ pkg.	220
Stroganoff	¼ pkg.	240
*(Lipton) & sauce:		
Regular:		
Beef	¼ pkg.	128
Chicken	¼ pkg.	190
Cheese	¼ pkg.	141

Food and Description	Measure or Quantity	Calories
Deluxe:		
Alfredo	¼ pkg.	146
Stroganoff	¼ pkg.	131
*NOODLE, RAMEN, canned (La Choy):		
Beef or oriental	1½ oz.	190
Chicken	1½ oz.	187
NOODLE, RICE (La Choy)	1 oz.	130
NOODLE ROMANOFF, frozen (Stouffer's)	⅓ pkg.	170
NOODLES & BEEF:		
Canned (Hormel) *Short Orders*	7½-oz. can	230
Frozen (Banquet) *Buffet Supper*	2-lb. pkg.	754
NOODLES & CHICKEN:		
Canned (Hormel) *Dinty Moore, Short Orders*	7½-oz. can	210
Frozen (Swanson)	10½-oz. dinner	270
NUT (See specific type: CASHEW, MACADAMIA, etc.)		
NUT, MIXED:		
Dry roasted:		
(Flavor House)	1 oz.	172
(Planters) salted	1 oz.	160
Honey roasted (Fisher)	1 oz.	150
Oil roasted (Planters) with or without peanuts	1 oz.	180
NUTMEG (French's)	1 tsp.	11
NUTRI-GRAIN, cereal (Kellogg's):		
Corn	½ cup	110
Wheat	⅔ cup	110
Wheat & Raisin	⅔ cup	140
NUTRIMATO (Mott's)	6 fl. oz.	70

O

Food and Description	Measure or Quantity	Calories
OAT FLAKES, cereal (Post)	⅔ cup	107
OATMEAL:		
Dry:		
Regular:		
(Elam's) Scotch style	1 oz.	108
(H-O) old fashioned	1 T.	15
(3-Minute Brand)	⅓ cup	110
Instant:		
(H-O):		
Regular, boxed	1 T.	15
With bran & spice	1½-oz. packet	157
With maple & brown sugar flavor	1½-oz. packet	160
(Quaker):		
Regular	1-oz. packet	105
Apple & cinnamon	1¼-oz. packet	134
Raisins & spice	1½-oz. packet	159
(3-Minute Brand)	½-oz. packet	162
Quick:		
(Harvest Brand)	⅓ cup	108
(Ralston Purina)	⅓ cup	110
(3-Minute Brand)	⅓ cup	110
Cooked, regular	1 cup	132
OIL, SALAD OR COOKING:		
(Bertoli) olive	1 T.	120
Crisco, Mazola	1 T.	126
Mrs. Tucker's; (Goya)	1 T.	130
Sunlite: Wesson	1 T.	120
OKRA, frozen:		
(Birds Eye) whole, baby	⅓ pkg.	36
(Frosty Acres):		
Cut	3.3 oz.	25
White	3.3 oz.	30
(Larsen) cut	3.3 oz.	25
(Seabrook Farms) cut	⅓ pkg.	32
(Southland) cut	⅕ of 16-oz. pkg.	30
OLD FASHIONED COCKTAIL		
(Hiram Walker) 62 proof	3 fl. oz.	165

Food and Description	Measure or Quantity	Calories
OLIVE:		
Green	4 med. or 3 extra large or 2 giant	19
Ripe, Mission	3 small or 2 large	18
OMELET, frozen (Swanson)		
TV Brand, Spanish style	7¾-oz. entree	240
ONION:		
Raw	2½" onion	38
Boiled, pearl onion	½ cup	27
Canned (Durkee) *O & C:*		
Boiled	¼ of 16-oz. jar.	32
Creamed	¼ of 15½-oz. can	554
Dehydrated (Gilroy) flakes	1 tsp.	5
Frozen:		
(Birds Eye):		
Creamed	⅓ pkg.	106
Whole, small	⅓ pkg.	44
(Frosty Acres) chopped	1 oz.	8
(Green Giant) in cheese sauce	½ cup	90
(Larsen):		
Diced	1 oz.	8
Whole	3.3 oz.	35
(Mrs. Paul's) french-fried rings	½ of 5-oz. pkg.	167
ONION BOUILLON:		
(Herb-Ox)	1 cube	10
MBT	1 packet	16
(Wyler's) instant	1 tsp.	10
ONION, COCKTAIL		
(Vlasic)	1 oz.	4
ONION, GREEN	1 small onion	4
ONION SALAD SEASONING		
(French's) instant	1 T.	15
ONION SALT (French's)	1 tsp.	6
ONION SOUP (See SOUP, Onion)		
ORANGE:		
Peeled	½ cup	62
Sections	4 oz.	58
ORANGE-APRICOT JUICE		
COCKTAIL, *Musselman's*	8 fl. oz.	100
ORANGE DRINK:		
Canned:		
Bama (Borden)	8.45-fl.-oz. container	120
Capri Sun	6¾-fl.-oz. can	103
(Hi-C)	8 fl. oz.	123
(Lincoln)	6 fl. oz.	90
Ssips (Johanna Farms)	8.45-fl.-oz. container	130
*Mix:		
Regular (Hi-C)	8 fl. oz.	91
Dietetic:		
Crystal Light	6 fl. oz.	4

Food and Description	Measure or Quantity	Calories
(Sunkist)	6 fl. oz.	6
ORANGE EXTRACT (Durkee) imitation	1 tsp.	15
ORANGE-GRAPEFRUIT JUICE:		
Canned (Libby's) unsweetened	6 fl. oz.	80
*Frozen (Minute Maid) unsweetened	6 fl. oz.	76
ORANGE JUICE:		
Canned:		
(Borden) Sippin' Pak	8.45-fl.-oz. container	110
(Del Monte) unsweetened	6 fl. oz.	80
(Johanna Farms)	6 fl. oz.	84
(Libby's) unsweetened	6 fl. oz.	90
(Texsun) sweetened	6 fl. oz.	83
Chilled (Sunkist)	6 fl. oz.	80
*Frozen:		
(Birds Eye) *Orange Plus*	6 fl. oz.	95
Bright & Early, imitation	6 fl. oz.	90
(Citrus Hill):		
Regular	6 fl. oz.	90
Lite	6 fl. oz.	60
(Sunkist)	6 fl. oz.	80
ORANGE JUICE BAR (Sunkist)	3-fl. oz. bar	70
ORANGE JUICE DRINK, canned (Sunkist)	8.45 fl. oz.	140
ORANGE PEEL, CANDIED	1 oz.	93
ORANGE-PINEAPPLE DRINK, canned (Lincoln)	6 fl. oz.	90
ORANGE-PINEAPPLE JUICE, canned (Texsun)	8 fl. oz.	89
ORCHARD BLEND JUICE, canned (Welch's):		
Apple-grape	6 fl. oz.	100
Harvest	6 fl. oz.	90
Vineyard	6 fl. oz.	120
OVALTINE, chocolate	¾ oz.	78
OVEN FRY (General Foods):		
Crispy crumb for pork	4.2-oz. envelope	484
Crispy crumb for chicken	4.2-oz. envelope	460
Homestyle flour recipe	3.2-oz. envelope	304
OYSTER:		
Raw:		
Eastern	19–31 small or 13–19 med.	158
Pacific & Western	6–9 small or 4–6 med.	218
Canned (Bumble Bee) shelled, whole, solids & liq.	1 cup	218
Fried	4 oz.	271
OYSTER STEW, home recipe	½ cup	103

P

Food and Description	Measure or Quantity	Calories
PAC-MAN, cereal (General Mills)	1 cup	110
***PANCAKE BATTER,** frozen (Aunt Jemima):		
Plain	4" pancake	70
Blueberry or buttermilk	4" pancake	68
PANCAKE DINNER OR ENTREE, frozen (Swanson):		
& blueberry sauce	7-oz. meal	400
& sausage	6-oz. meal	460
PANCAKE & SAUSAGE, frozen (Swanson)	6-oz. entree	440
***PANCAKE & WAFFLE MIX:**		
Plain:		
(Aunt Jemima) Original	4" pancake	73
(Log Cabin) Complete	4" pancake	58
(Pillsbury) *Hungry Jack:*		
Complete, bulk	4" pancake	63
Extra Lights	4" pancake	70
Golden Blend, complete	4" pancake	80
Panshakes	4" pancake	83
Blueberry (Pillsbury) *Hungry Jack*	4" pancake	107
Buckwheat (Aunt Jemima)	4" pancake	67
Buttermilk:		
(Aunt Jemima) regular	4" pancake	100
(Betty Crocker) complete	4" pancake	70
(Pillsbury) *Hungry Jack,* complete	4" pancake	63
Whole wheat (Aunt Jemima)	4" pancake	83
Dietetic:		
(Estee)	3" pancake	33
(Featherweight)	4" pancake	43
PANCAKE & WAFFLE SYRUP (See SYRUP, Pancake & Waffle)		
PAPAYA, fresh:		
Cubed	½ cup	36
Juice	4 oz.	78
PAPRIKA (French's)	1 tsp.	7
PARSLEY:		
Fresh, chopped	1 T.	2
Dried (French's)	1 tsp.	4

Food and Description	Measure or Quantity	Calories
PASSION FRUIT, giant, whole	1 lb.	53
PASTINAS, egg	1 oz.	109
PASTRAMI (Carl Buddig)	1 oz.	40
PASTRY POCKETS (Pillsbury)	1 pocket	230
PASTRY SHEET, PUFF, frozen (Pepperidge Farm)	1 sheet	1150
PÂTÉ:		
De foie gras	1 T.	69
Liver:		
(Hormel)	1 T.	35
(Sell's)	1 T.	93
PDQ:		
Chocolate	1 T.	66
Strawberry	1 T.	60
PEA, green:		
Boiled	½ cup	58
Canned, regular pack, solids & liq.:		
(Comstock)	½ cup	70
(Del Monte) seasoned or sweet, regular size	½ cup	60
(Green Giant):		
Early with onions, sweet or sweet with onions	¼ of 17-oz. can	60
Sweet, mini	¼ of 17-oz. can	64
(Larsen) *Fresh-Lite*	½ cup	50
Canned, dietetic pack, solids & liq.:		
(Del Monte) no salt added, sweet	½ cup	60
(Diet Delight)	½ cup	50
(Featherweight) sweet	½ cup	70
(Larsen) *Fresh-Lite,* low sodium	½ cup	50
Frozen:		
(Birds Eye):		
Regular	⅓ pkg.	78
In butter sauce	⅓ pkg.	85
In cream sauce	⅓ pkg.	84
(Frosty Acres):		
Regular	3.3 oz.	80
Tiny	3.3 oz.	60
(Green Giant):		
In cream sauce	½ cup	100
Sweet, *Harvest Fresh*	½ cup	80
PEA & CARROT:		
Canned, regular pack, solids & liq.:		
(Comstock)	½ cup	60
(Del Monte)	½ cup	50
(Libby's)	½ cup	56
(Veg-All)	½ cup	50

Food and Description	Measure or Quantity	Calories
Canned, dietetic pack, solids & liq.:		
(Diet Delight)	½ cup	40
(Larsen) *Fresh-Lite*, low sodium	½ cup	50
(S&W) *Nutradiet*	½ cup	35
Frozen:		
(Birds Eye)	⅓ pkg.	61
(Larsen)	3.3 oz.	60
(McKenzie)	3.3-oz. serving	60
PEA, CROWDER, frozen		
(Southland)	⅓ of 16-oz. pkg.	130
PEA POD:		
Boiled, drained solids	4 oz.	49
Frozen (La Choy)	6-oz. pkg.	70
PEACH:		
Fresh, with thin skin	2″ dia.	38
Fresh slices	½ cup	32
Canned, regular pack, solids & liq.:		
(Del Monte) Cling:		
Halves or slices	½ cup	80
Spiced	3½ oz.	80
(Hunt's) *Snack Pack*	5-oz. container	110
(Libby's) heavy syrup:		
Halves	½ cup	105
Sliced	½ cup	102
Canned, dietetic pack, solids & liq.:		
(Del Monte) Lite, Cling	½ cup	50
(Diet Delight) Cling:		
Juice pack	½ cup	50
Water Pack	½ cup	30
(Featherweight);		
Cling or Freestone, juice pack	½ cup	50
Cling, water pack	½ cup	30
(S&W) *Nutradiet,* Cling:		
Juice pack	½ cup	60
Water pack	½ cup	30
Frozen (Birds Eye)	5-oz. pkg.	141
PEACH BUTTER (Smucker's)	1 T.	45
PEACH DRINK, canned (Hi-C):		
Canned	6 fl.oz.	90
*Mix	6 fl. oz.	72
PEACH LIQUEUR (DeKuyper)	1 fl. oz.	82
PEACH NECTAR, canned (Libby's)	6 fl. oz.	90
PEACH PRESERVE OR JAM:		
Sweetened:		
(Bama)	1 T.	45
(Home Brands)	1 T.	50
(Smucker's)	1 T.	53
Dietetic (Dia-Mel)	1 T.	6

Food and Description	Measure or Quantity	Calories
PEANUT:		
In shell (Planters)	1 oz.	160
Dry roasted:		
(Fisher)	1 oz.	163
(Planters)	1 oz.	160
(Tom's)	1 oz.	160
Honey roasted:		
(Eagle)	1 oz.	170
(Fisher)	1 oz.	150
Oil roasted (Planters) salted	1 oz.	170
PEANUT BUTTER:		
Regular:		
(Adams)	1 T.	95
(Bama) creamy or crunchy	1 T.	100
(Elam's) natural	1 T.	109
(Holsum)	1 T.	94
(Home Brands)	1 T.	105
(Laura Scudder's)	1 T.	95
(Peter Pan)	1 T.	90
(Skippy) creamy or super chunk	1 T.	108
Dietetic:		
(Adams) low sodium	1 T.	95
(Home Brands):		
Lightly salted or unsalted	1 T.	105
No sugar added	1 T.	90
(Peter Pan) creamy	1 T.	95
(S&W) *Nutradiet,* low sodium	1 T.	93
(Smucker's) low sodium	1 T.	100
PEANUT BUTTER BAKING		
CHIPS (Reese's)	3 T. (1 oz.)	153
PEANUT BUTTER & JELLY (Bama)	1 T.	75
PEAR:		
Whole	3″ × 2½″ pear	101
Canned, regular pack, solids & liq.:		
(Del Monte) Bartlett	½ cup	80
(Libby's)	½ cup	102
Canned, dietetic pack, solids & liq.:		
(Del Monte) Lite	½ cup	50
(Featherweight) Bartlett:		
Juice pack	½ cup	60
Water pack	½ cup	40
(Libby's) water pack	½ cup	60
Dried (Sun-Maid)	½ cup	260
PEAR-APPLE JUICE (Tree Top)	6 fl. oz.	90
PEAR-GRAPE JUICE (Tree Top)	6 fl. oz.	100
PEAR NECTAR, canned (Libby's)	6 fl. oz.	100
PEAR-PASSION FRUIT NECTAR,		
canned (Libby's)	6 fl. oz.	60

Food and Description	Measure or Quantity	Calories
PEAR, STRAINED		
(Larsen)	½ cup	65
PEBBLES, cereal:		
Cocoa	⅞ cup	117
Fruity	⅞ cup	116
PECAN:		
Halves	6-7 pieces	48
Roasted, dry:		
(Fisher) salted	1 oz.	220
(Planters)	1 oz.	190
PECTIN, FRUIT:		
Certo	6-oz. pkg.	19
Sure-Jell	1¾-oz. pkg.	170
PEPPER:		
Black (French's)	1 tsp.	9
Seasoned (French's)	1 tsp.	8
PEPPER & ONION, frozen		
(Southland)	2-oz. serving	15
PEPPER, BANANA (Vlasic)		
hot rings	1 oz.	4
PEPPER, CHERRY (Vlasic) mild	1 oz.	8
PEPPER, CHILI, canned:		
(Del Monte):		
Green, whole	½ cup	20
Jalapeño or chili, whole	½ cup	30
Old El Paso, green, chopped		
or whole	1 oz.	7
(Ortega):		
Diced, strips or whole	1 oz.	10
Jalapeño, diced or whole	1 oz.	9
(Vlasic) Jalapeño	1 oz.	8
PEPPERMINT EXTRACT (Durkee)		
imitation	1 tsp.	15
PEPPERONCINI (Vlasic)		
Greek, mild	1 oz.	4
PEPPERONI:		
(Eckrich)	1-oz. serving	135
(Hormel) regular or Rosa Grande	1-oz. serving	140
PEPPER STEAK:		
*Canned (La Choy)	¾ cup	210
Frozen:		
(Blue Star) *Dining Lite,* with rice	9½-oz. entree	267
(Le Menu)	11½-oz. dinner	360
(Stouffer's)	5¼-oz. serving	354
PEPPER, STUFFED:		
Home recipe	2¾" × 2½" pepper with 1⅛ cups stuffing	314
Frozen:		
(Celentano)	12½-oz. pkg.	290

Food and Description	Measure or Quantity	Calories
(Stouffer's) green	7¾-oz. serving	225
(Weight Watchers) with veal stuffing	11¾-oz. meal	270
PEPPER, SWEET:		
Raw:		
Green:		
Whole	1 lb.	82
Without stem & seeds	1 med. pepper (2.6 oz.)	13
Red:		
Whole	1 lb.	112
Without stem & seeds	1 med. pepper (2.2 oz.)	19
Boiled, green, without salt, drained	1 med. pepper (2.6 oz.)	13
Frozen:		
(Frosty Acres) diced:		
Green	1 oz.	6
Red & green	1 oz.	7
(Larsen) green	1 oz.	6
(McKenzie)	1-oz. serving	6
(Southland) diced	2-oz. serving	10
PERCH, OCEAN:		
Atlantic, raw:		
Whole	1 lb.	124
Meat only	4 oz.	108
Pacific, raw, whole	1 lb.	116
Frozen:		
(Banquet)	8¾-oz. dinner	434
(Frionor) *Norway Gourmet*	4 oz. fillet	120
(Mrs. Paul's) fillet, breaded & fried	2-oz. piece	145
(Van de Kamp's) batter dipped, french fried	2-oz. piece	135
PERNOD (Julius Wile)	1 fl. oz.	79
PERSIMMON:		
Japanese or Kaki, fresh:		
With seeds	4.4-oz. piece	79
Seedless	4.4-oz. piece	81
Native, fresh, flesh only	4-oz. serving	144
PETITE SIRAH WINE (Louis M. Martini):		
Regular, 12% alcohol	3 fl. oz.	62
White, 12.3% alcohol	3 fl. oz.	54
PHEASANT, raw, meat only	4-oz. serving	184
PICKLE:		
Cucumber, fresh or bread & butter:		
(Fannings)	1.2-oz. serving	17
(Featherweight) low sodium	1-oz. pickle	12

Food and Description	Measure or Quantity	Calories
(Vlasic):		
Chips	1 oz.	7
Stix, sweet butter	1 oz.	5
Dill:		
(Featherweight) low sodium, whole	1-oz. serving	4
(Smucker's):		
Hamburger, sliced	1 slice	Tr.
Polish, whole	3½" pickle	8
(Vlasic):		
Original	1 oz.	2
No garlic	1 oz.	4
Hamburger (Vlasic) chips	1-oz. serving	2
Hot & spicy (Vlasic) garden mix	1 oz.	4
Kosher dill:		
(Claussen) halves or whole	2-oz. serving	7
(Featherweight) low sodium	1-oz. serving	4
(Smucker's):		
Baby	2¾"-long pickle	4
Whole	3½"-long pickle	8
(Vlasic)	1 oz.	4
Sweet:		
(Nalley's) *Nubbins*	1-oz. serving	28
(Smucker's):		
Gherkins	2"-long pickle	15
Whole	2½"-long pickle	18
(Vlasic)	1 oz.	30
Sweet & sour (Claussen) slices	1 slice	3
PIE:		
Regular, non-frozen:		
Apple:		
Home recipe, two crust	⅙ of 9" pie	404
(Hostess)	4½-oz. pie	390
Banana, home recipe, cream or custard	⅙ of 9" pie	336
Berry (Hostess)	4½-oz. pie	404
Blackberry, home recipe, two-crust	⅙ of 9" pie	384
Blueberry:		
Home recipe, two-crust	⅙ of 9" pie	382
(Hostess)	4½-oz. pie	394
Boston cream, home recipe	1/12 of 8" pie	208
Butterscotch, home recipe, one-crust	⅙ of 9" pie	406
Cherry:		
Home recipe, two-crust	⅙ of 9" pie	412
(Hostess)	4½-oz. pie	390
Chocolate chiffon, home recipe	⅙ of 9" pie	459
Chocolate meringue, home recipe	⅙ of 9"pie	353

Food and Description	Measure or Quantity	Calories
Coconut custard, home recipe	⅙ of 9"pie	357
Lemon (Hostess)	4½-oz. pie	400
Lemon meringue, home recipe, one-crust	⅙ of 9" pie	357
Mince, home recipe, two-crust	⅙ of 9" pie	428
Peach (Hostess)	4½-oz. pie	400
Pumpkin, home recipe, one-crust	⅙ of 9" pie	321
Raisin, home recipe, two-crust	⅙ of 9" pie	427
Strawberry (Hostess)	4½-oz. pie	340
Frozen:		
Apple:		
(Banquet) family size	⅙ of 20-oz. pie	253
(Morton):		
Regular	⅙ of 24-oz. pie	296
Great Little Desserts, regular	8-oz. pie	590
(Weight Watchers)	3 oz.	180
Banana cream:		
(Banquet)	⅙ of 14-oz. pie	172
(Morton) regular	⅙ of 16-oz. pie	174
Blackberry (Banquet)	⅙ of 20-oz. pie	268
Blueberry:		
(Banquet)	⅙ of 20-oz. pie	266
(Morton) *Great Little Desserts*	8-oz. pie	580
Cherry:		
(Banquet)	⅙ of 20-oz. pie	252
(Morton) regular	⅙ of 24-oz. pie	300
(Weight Watchers)	3 oz.	200
Chocolate (Morton)	⅙ of 14-oz. pie	180
Chocolate cream:		
(Banquet)	⅙ of 14-oz. pie	177
(Morton) *Great Little Desserts*	3½-oz. pie	270
Coconut cream (Banquet)	⅙ of 14-oz. pie	179
Coconut custard (Morton)		
Great Little Desserts	6½-oz. pie	370
Lemon cream:		
(Banquet)	⅙ of 14-oz. pie	168
(Morton) *Great Little Desserts*	3½-oz. pie	250
Mince:		
(Banquet)	⅙ of 20-oz. pie	258
(Morton)	⅙ of 24-oz. pie	310
Peach (Sara Lee)	⅙ of 31-oz. pie	458
Pumpkin:		
(Banquet)	⅙ of 20-oz. pie	197
(Morton) regular	⅙ of 24-oz. pie	230
Strawberry cream (Banquet)	⅙ of 14-oz. pie	168
PIECRUST:		
Home recipe, 9" pie	1 crust	900
Refrigerated (Pillsbury)	2 crusts	1920

Food and Description	Measure or Quantity	Calories
*PIECRUST MIX:		
(Betty Crocker):		
Regular	1/16 pkg.	120
Stick	1/8 stick	120
(Flako)	1/6 of 9" pie shell	245
(Pillsbury) mix or stick	1/6 of 2-crust pie	270
PIE FILLING (See also PUDDING OR PIE FILLING):		
Apple:		
(Comstock)	1/6 of 21-oz. can	110
(Thank You Brand)	3½ oz.	91
Apple rings or slices (See APPLE, canned)		
Apricot (Comstock)	1/6 of 21-oz. can	110
Banana cream (Comstock)	1/6 of 21-oz. can	110
Blueberry (Comstock)	1/6 of 21-oz. can	120
Cherry (Thank You Brand) regular	3½ oz.	99
Coconut cream (Comstock)	1/6 of 21-oz. can	120
Coconut custard, home recipe, made with egg yolk & milk	5 oz. (inc. crust)	288
Lemon (Comstock)	1/6 of 21-oz. can	160
Mincemeat (Comstock)	½ of 21-oz. can	170
Pumpkin (Libby's) (See also PUMPKIN, canned)	1 cup	210
Raisin (Comstock)	1/6 of 21-oz. can	140
*PIE MIX:		
Boston Cream (Betty Crocker)	1/8 of pie	260
Chocolate (Royal)	1/8 of pie	260
PIEROGIES, frozen:		
(Empire Kosher):		
Cheese	1½ oz.	110
Onion	1½ oz.	90
(Mrs. Paul's) potato & cheese	1 piece	90
PIGS FEET, pickled	4-oz. serving	226
PIMIENTO, canned:		
(Dromedary) drained	1-oz. serving	10
(Ortega)	¼ cup	6
(Sunshine) diced or sliced	1 T.	4
PIÑA COLADA (Mr. Boston) 12½% alcohol	3 fl. oz.	249
*PIÑA COLADA MIX		
(Bar-Tender's)	5 fl. oz.	254
PINEAPPLE:		
Fresh, chunks	½ cup	52
Canned, regular pack, solids & liq.:		
(Del Monte) slices, syrup pack	½ cup	90
(Dole):		
Juice pack, chunk, crushed or sliced	½ cup	70

Food and Description	Measure or Quantity	Calories
Heavy syrup, chunk, crushed or sliced	½ cup	95
Canned, unsweetened or dietetic, solids & liq.:		
(Diet Delight) juice pack	½ cup	70
(Libby's) Lite	½ cup	60
(S&W) *Nutradiet*	1 slice	30
PINEAPPLE & GRAPEFRUIT JUICE DRINK, canned:		
(Del Monte) regular or pink	6 fl. oz.	90
(Dole) pink	6 fl. oz.	101
(Texsun)	6 fl. oz.	91
PINEAPPLE, CANDIED	1-oz. serving	90
PINEAPPLE FLAVORING (Durkee) imitation	1 tsp.	6
PINEAPPLE JUICE:		
Canned:		
(Del Monte)	6 fl. oz.	100
(Dole)	6 fl. oz.	103
(Texsun)	6 fl. oz.	97
*Frozen (Minute Maid)	6 fl. oz.	92
PINEAPPLE-ORANGE DRINK, canned (Hi-C)	6 fl. oz.	94
PINEAPPLE-ORANGE JUICE:		
Canned:		
(Del Monte)	6 fl. oz.	90
(Johanna Farms) *Tree Ripe*	8.45-fl.-oz. container	132
*Frozen (Minute Maid)	6 fl. oz.	94
PINEAPPLE PRESERVE OR JAM, sweetened (Home Brands)	1 T.	52
PINE NUT, pignolias, shelled	1 oz.	156
PINOT CHARDONNAY WINE (Paul Masson) 12% alcohol	3 fl. oz.	71
PISTACHIO NUT:		
In shell	½ cup	197
Shelled	¼ cup	184
(Fisher) shelled, roasted, salted	1 oz.	174
PIZZA PIE (See also **SHAKEY'S**):		
Regular, non-frozen:		
Home recipe	⅛ of 14" pie	177
(*Domino's*):		
Beef, ground:		
Plain:		
12" pizza (small)	1 slice	216
16" pizza (large)	1 slice	303
With pepperoni:		
12" pizza (small)	1 slice	216
16" pizza (large)	1 slice	303

Food and Description	Measure or Quantity	Calories
Cheese:		
Plain:		
12" pizza (small)	1 slice	157
16" pizza (large)	1 slice	239
Double cheese:		
12" pizza (small)	1 slice	240
16" pizza (large)	1 slice	350
Double, with pepperoni		
12" pizza (small)	1 slice	227
16" pizza (large)	1 slice	389
Mushroom & sausage:		
12" pizza (small)	1 slice	183
16" pizza (large)	1 slice	266
Pepperoni:		
Plain:		
12" pizza (small)	1 slice	192
16" pizza (large)	1 slice	278
With mushrooms:		
12" pizza (small)	1 slice	194
16" pizza (large)	1 slice	280
With sausage:		
12" pizza (small)	1 slice	215
16" pizza (large)	1 slice	303
Sausage:		
12" pizza (small)	1 slice	180
16" pizza (large)	1 slice	264
(Godfather's):		
Cheese:		
Original:		
Mini	¼ of 11-oz. piece	190
Medium	⅛ of 32-oz. pie	270
Stuffed, medium	⅛ of 38-oz. pie	350
Trim crust, large	1/10 of 34-oz. pie	228
Combo:		
Original:		
Hot slice	1/10 of 67-oz. pie	437
Small	⅙ of 33-oz. pie	360
Stuffed, medium	⅛ of 56-oz. pie	480
Thin crust, small	⅙ of 26-oz. pie	270
Frozen:		
Canadian style bacon (Celeste)	8-oz. pie	483
Cheese:		
(Celentano):		
Mini slice	1 slice	157
Thick crust	⅓ of 13-oz. pie	238
(Stouffer's) French Bread	½ of 10⅜-oz. pkg.	330
(Weight Watchers)	6-oz. pie	350
Combination:		
(Celeste) Chicago style	¼ of 24-oz. pie	360

Food and Description	Measure or Quantity	Calories
(La Pizzeria)	½ of 13½-oz. pie	420
(Van de Kamp's) thick crust	¼ of 24½-oz. pie	310
(Weight Watchers)	7¼-oz. pie	322
Deluxe:		
(Celeste)	½ of 9-oz. pie	281
(Stouffer's) French Bread	½ of 12⅜-oz. pkg.	400
Hamburger (Stouffer's) French Bread	½ of 12¼-oz. pkg.	400
Mushroom (Stouffer's) French Bread	½ of 12-oz. pkg.	340
Pepperoni:		
(Stouffer's) French Bread	½ of 11¼-oz. pkg.	410
(Weight Watchers)	6¼-oz. pie	370
Sausage:		
(Celeste)	½ of 8-oz. pie	262
(Stouffer's) French Bread	½ of 12-oz. pkg.	420
(Weight Watchers) veal	6¾-oz. pie	350
Sausage & mushroom:		
(Celeste)	¼ of 24-oz. pie	365
(Stouffer's) French Bread	½ of 12½-oz. pkg.	395
Sicilian style (Celeste) deluxe	¼ of 26-oz. pie	408
Supreme (Celeste) without meat	½ of 8-oz. pie	217
*Mix (Ragú) *Pizza Quick*	¼ of pie	300
PIZZA PIE CRUST, refrigerated (Pillsbury)	⅛ of crust	90
PIZZA SAUCE:		
(Contadina):		
Regular or with cheese	½ cup	80
With pepperoni	½ cup	90
(Ragú):		
Regular	2 oz.	32
Pizza Quick	2 oz.	45
PLUM:		
Fresh, Japanese & hybrid	2″ dia.	27
Fresh, prune-type, halves	½ cup	60
Canned, regular pack:		
(Stokely-Van Camp)	½ cup	120
(Thank You Brand) heavy syrup	½ cup	109
Canned, unsweetened, purple, solids & liq.:		
(Diet Delight) juice pack	½ cup	70
(Featherweight) water pack	½ cup	40
(S&W) *Nutradiet,* juice pack	½ cup	80
PLUM JELLY, sweetened (Home Brands)	1 T.	52
PLUM PRESERVE OR JAM, sweetened (Bama)	1 T.	45
PLUM PUDDING (Richardson & Robbins)	2″ wedge	270

Food and Description	Measure or Quantity	Calories
POLYNESIAN-STYLE DINNER,		
frozen (Swanson)	12-oz. dinner	360
POMEGRANATE, whole	1 lb.	160
PONDEROSA RESTAURANT:		
A-1 Sauce	1 tsp.	4
Beef, chopped (patty only):		
Regular	3½ oz.	209
Double Deluxe	5.9 oz.	362
Junior (*Square Shooter*)	1.6 oz.	98
Steakhouse Deluxe	2.96 oz.	181
Beverages:		
Coca-Cola	8 fl. oz.	96
Coffee	6 fl. oz.	2
Dr. Pepper	8 fl. oz.	96
Milk, chocolate	8 fl. oz.	208
Orange drink	8 fl. oz.	110
Root beer	8 fl. oz.	104
Sprite	8 fl. oz.	95
Tab	8 fl. oz.	1
Bun:		
Regular	2.4-oz. bun	190
Hot dog	1 bun	108
Junior	1.4-oz. bun	118
Steakhouse deluxe	2.4-oz. bun	190
Chicken strips:		
Adult portion	2¾ oz.	282
Child	1.4 oz.	141
Cocktail sauce	1½ oz.	57
Filet mignon	3.8 oz. (edible portion)	57
Filet of sole, fish only (See also Bun: regualar)	3-oz. piece	125
Fish, baked	4.9-oz. serving	268
Gelatin dessert	½ cup	97
Gravy, au jus	1 oz.	3
Ham & cheese:		
Bun (see Bun)		
Cheese, Swiss	2 slices (.8 oz.)	76
Ham	2½ oz.	184
Hot dog, child's, meat only (see also Bun)	1.6-oz. hot dog	140
Margarine:		
Pat	1 tsp.	36
On potato, as served	½ oz.	100
Mustard sauce, sweet & sour	1 oz.	50
New York strip steak	6.1 oz. (edible portion)	362
Onion, chopped	1 T.	4
Pickle, dill	3 slices (.7 oz.)	2

Food and Description	Measure or Quantity	Calories
Potato:		
Baked	7.2-oz. potato	145
French fries	3-oz. serving	230
Prime ribs:		
Regular	4.2 oz. (edible portion)	286
King	6 oz. (edible portion)	409
Pudding, chocolate	4½ oz.	213
Ribeye	3.2 oz. (edible portion)	197
Ribeye & shrimp:		
Ribeye	3.2 oz.	197
Shrimp	2.2 oz.	139
Roll, kaiser	2.2-oz. roll	184
Salad bar:		
Bean sprouts	1 oz.	13
Broccoli	1 oz.	9
Cabbage, red	1 oz.	9
Carrots	1 oz.	12
Cauliflower	1 oz.	8
Celery	1 oz.	4
Chickpeas (Garbanzos)	1 oz.	102
Mushrooms	1 oz.	8
Pepper, green	1 oz.	6
Radish	1 oz.	5
Tomato	1 oz.	6
Salad dressing:		
Blue cheese	1 oz.	129
Italian, creamy	1 oz.	138
Low calorie	1 oz.	14
Oil & vinegar	1 oz.	124
Thousand Island	1 oz.	117
Shrimp dinner	7 pieces (3½ oz.)	220
Sirloin:		
Regular	3.3 oz. (edible portion)	220
Super	6½ oz. (edible portion)	383
Tips	4 oz. (edible portion)	192
Steak sauce	1 oz.	23
Tartar sauce	1.5 oz.	285
T-Bone	4.3 oz. (edible portion)	240
Tomato (See also Salad bar):		
Slices	2 slices (.9 oz.)	5
Whole, small	3.5 oz.	22
Topping, whipped	¼ oz.	19

Food and Description	Measure or Quantity	Calories
Worcestershire sauce	1 tsp.	4
POPCORN:		
*Plain, popped fresh:		
(Jiffy Pop)	½ of 5-oz. pkg.	244
(Jolly Time) white	1 cup	19
(Orville Reddenbacher's) Gourmet Original:		
Plain	1 cup	22
With oil & salt	1 cup	40
Caramel crunch	1 oz.	140
Hot air popped	1 cup	25
Microwave:		
Regular:		
Butter flavored	1 cup	27
Natural	1 cup	27
Flavored:		
Caramel	1 cup	96
Cheese, cheddar	1 cup	50
Frozen	1 cup	35
(Pillsbury) Microwave Popcorn:		
Regular	1 cup	70
Butter flavor	1 cup	65
Packaged:		
Buttered (Wise)	½ oz.	70
Caramel-coated:		
(Bachman)	1-oz. serving	130
(Old London) without peanuts	1¾-oz. serving	195
Cheese flavored (Bachman)	1-oz. serving	180
Cracker Jack	1-oz. serving	120
POPCORN POPPING OIL (Orville Reddenbacher's) buttery flavor	1 T.	120
***POPOVER MIX** (Flako)	1 popover	170
POPPY SEED (French's)	1 tsp.	13
***POPSICLE,** twin pop	3 fl. oz.	70
POP TARTS (See TOASTER CAKE OR PASTRY)		
PORK:		
Fresh:		
Chop:		
Broiled, lean & fat	3-oz. chop (weighed without bone)	332
Broiled, lean only	3-oz. chop (weighed without bone)	230
Loin:		
Roasted, lean & fat	3 oz.	308
Roasted, lean only	3 oz.	216
Spareribs, braised	3 oz.	246
Cured ham:		
Roasted, lean & fat	3 oz.	246

Food and Description	Measure or Quantity	Calories
Roasted, lean only	3 oz.	159
PORK DINNER: frozen (Swanson)	11¼-oz. dinner	290
PORK DINNER OR ENTREE:		
Canned (Hunt's) *Minute Gourmet Microwave Entree Maker,* cajun:		
Without pork	3.9 oz.	180
*With pork	6.6 oz.	460
Frozen (Swanson) dinner, loin of	11¼-oz. dinner	290
PORK, PACKAGED (Eckrich)	1-oz. serving	45
PORK RINDS (Tom's)	.6 oz. serving	60
PORK STEAK, BREADED, frozen (Hormel)	3-oz. serving	223
PORK, SWEET & SOUR, frozen (La Choy)	½ of 15-oz. pkg.	229
PORT WINE:		
(Gallo)	3 fl. oz.	94
(Louis M. Martini)	3 fl. oz.	82
POSTUM, instant	6 fl. oz.	11
POTATO:		
Cooked:		
Au gratin	½ cup	127
Baked, peeled	2½″-dia. potato	92
Boiled, peeled	4.2-oz. potato	79
French-fried	10 pieces	156
Hash-browned, home recipe	½ cup	223
Mashed, milk & butter added	½ cup	92
Canned, solids & liq.:		
(Allen's) *Butterfield*	½ cup	45
(Del Monte)	½ cup (4 oz.)	45
(Larsen) *Freshlike,* sliced or whole	½ cup (4.5 oz.)	61
Frozen:		
(Birds Eye):		
Cottage fries	2.8-oz. serving	119
Crinkle cuts, regular	3-oz. serving	115
Farm style wedge	3-oz. serving	109
French fries, regular	3-oz. serving	113
Hash browns, shredded	¼ of 12-oz. pkg.	61
Steak fries	3-oz. serving	109
Tasti Puffs	¼ of 10-oz. pkg.	192
Tiny Taters	⅕ of 16-oz. pkg.	204
Whole, peeled	3.2 oz.	59
(Empire Kosher) french fries	3 oz.	110
(Green Giant):		
Sliced, in butter sauce	½ cup	80
& sweet peas in bacon cream sauce	½ cup	110
(Larsen) diced	4 oz.	80
(Stouffer's):		
Au gratin	⅓ pkg.	135

Food and Description	Measure or Quantity	Calories
Scalloped	⅓ pkg.	125
POTATO & BACON, canned		
(Hormel) *Short Orders*, au gratin	7½-oz. can	240
POTATO & BEEF, canned,		
Dinty Moore (Hormel) *Short Orders*	1½-oz. can	250
POTATO & HAM, canned (Hormel)		
Short Orders, scalloped	7½-oz. can	250
POTATO CHIP:		
(Cottage Fries) unsalted	1 oz.	160
(Featherweight) unsalted	1 oz.	160
(Frito-Lay's) natural	1 oz.	157
(Laura Scudder's)	1 oz.	150
Lay's, sour cream & onion flavor	1 oz.	160
(New York Deli)	1 oz.	160
O'Grady's	1 oz.	150
Pringle's:		
Regular or *Cheez-Ums*	1 oz.	167
Light	1 oz.	148
(Snyder's)	1 oz.	150
Ruffles, regular	1 oz.	150
(Tom's) any type	1 oz.	160
(Wise):		
Barbecue or garlic & onion	1 oz.	150
Lightly salted, natural or		
salt & vinegar	1 oz.	160
*POTATO MIX:		
Au gratin:		
(Betty Crocker)	½ cup	150
(French's) tangy	½ cup	130
(Libby's) *Potato Classics*	¾ cup	130
Creamed (Betty Crocker)	½ cup	160
Hash browns (Betty Crocker)		
with onion	½ cup	150
Hickory smoke cheese		
(Betty Crocker)	½ cup	150
Julienne (Betty Crocker) with mild		
cheese sauce	½ cup	130
Mashed:		
(Betty Crocker) *Buds*	½ cup	130
(French's)	½ cup	140
Scalloped:		
(Betty Crocker)	½ cup	140
(Libby's) *Potato Classics*	¾ cup	130
Sour cream & chive (Betty Crocker)	½ cup	150
*POTATO PANCAKE MIX		
(French's)	3" pancake	43
POTATO SALAD:		
Home recipe	½ cup	181
Canned (Nalley's) German style	4-oz. serving	143

Food and Description	Measure or Quantity	Calories
POTATO STARCH		
(Manischewitz) pure	½ cup	315
POTATO STICKS (Durkee) *O & C*	1½-oz. can	231
POTATO, STUFFED, BAKED, frozen (Green Giant):		
With cheese flavored topping	½ of 10-oz. pkg.	200
With sour cream & chives	½ of 10-oz. pkg.	230
POTATO TOPPERS (Libby's)	1 T.	30
POUND CAKE (See CAKE, Pound)		
PRESERVE OR JAM (See individual flavors)		
PRETZEL:		
(Eagle Snacks)	1 oz.	110
(Estee) unsalted	1 piece	5
(Nabisco) *Mister Salty:*		
Dutch	1 piece	55
Mini	1 piece	7
Nuggets	1 piece	5
Twists	1 piece	22
(Rokeach)	1 oz.	110
Rold Gold	1 oz.	110
(Snyder's) hard	1 oz.	102
(Tom's) twists	1 oz.	100
(Wise) nugget	1 oz.	110
PRODUCT 19, cereal (Kellogg's)	1 cup	110
PROSCIUTTO (Hormel) boneless	1 oz.	90
PRUNE:		
Canned:		
(Featherweight) stewed, water pack	½ cup	130
(Sunsweet) stewed	½ cup	120
Dried:		
(Del Monte) Moist Pak	2 oz.	120
(Sunsweet) whole	2 oz.	130
PRUNE JUICE:		
(Del Monte)	6 fl. oz.	120
(Mott's) regular	6 fl. oz.	140
(Sunsweet) regular	6 fl. oz.	140
PRUNE NECTAR, canned (Mott's)	6 fl. oz.	100
PUDDING OR PIE FILLING:		
Canned, regular pack:		
Banana:		
(Del Monte) *Pudding Cup*	5-oz. container	181
(Hunt's) *Snack Pack*	4¼-oz. container	180
(Thank You Brand)	½ cup	150
Butterscotch:		
(Del Monte) *Pudding Cup*	5-oz. container	184
(Swiss Miss)	4-oz. container	160
(Thank You Brand)	½ cup	149

Food and Description	Measure or Quantity	Calories
Chocolate:		
(Del Monte) *Pudding Cup*	5-oz. container	201
(Hunt's) *Snack Pack*, regular	4¼-oz. container	180
(Swiss Miss) fudge or fruit on		
bottom	4-oz. container	170
(Thank You Brand)	½ cup	191
Rice (Comstock; Menner's)	½ of 7½-oz. can	120
Tapioca:		
(Del Monte) *Pudding Cup*	5-oz. container	172
(Hunt's) *Snack Pack*	4¼-oz. container	140
Vanilla (Del Monte)	5-oz. container	188
Canned, dietetic pack:		
(Estee)	½ cup	70
(Sego)	4-oz. serving	125
Chilled, *Swiss Miss:*		
Butterscotch, chocolate malt		
or vanilla	4-oz. container	150
Chocolate or double rich	4-oz. container	160
Tapioca	4-oz. container	130
Frozen (Rich's):		
Banana	3-oz. container	142
Butterscotch or vanilla	4½-oz. container	199
Chocolate	4½-oz. container	214
*Mix, sweetened, regular & instant:		
Banana:		
(Jello-O) cream, regular	½ cup	161
(Royal) regular	½ cup	160
Butter pecan (Jello-O) instant	½ cup	175
Butterscotch:		
(Jell-O) instant	½ cup	175
(My-T-Fine) regular	½ cup	143
Chocolate:		
(Jell-O) regular	½ cup	174
(My-T-Fine) regular	½ cup	169
Coconut:		
(Jell-O) cream, regular	½ cup	176
(Royal) instant	½ cup	170
Flan (Royal) regular	½ cup	150
Lemon:		
(Jell-O) instant	½ cup	170
(My-T-Fine) regular	½ cup	164
Lime (Royal) Key Lime, regular	½ cup	160
Pineapple (Jell-O) cream, instant	½ cup	176
Pistachio (Jell-O) instant	½ cup	174
Raspberry (Salada)		
Danish Dessert	½ cup	176
Rice, *Jell-O Americana*	½ cup	176
Strawberry (Salada)		
Danish Dessert	½ cup	130

Food and Description	Measure or Quantity	Calories
Tapioca:		
Jell-O Americana, chocolate	½ cup	173
(My-T-Fine) vanilla	½ cup	130
Vanilla:		
(Jell-O) French, regular	½ cup	172
(Royal)	½ cup	180
*Mix, dietetic:		
Butterscotch:		
(D-Zerta)	½ cup	68
(Featherweight) artificially sweetened	½ cup	60
(Royal) instant	½ cup	100
Chocolate:		
(Dia-Mel)	½ cup	50
(Estee)	½ cup	70
(Royal) instant	½ cup	100
Lemon:		
(Dia-Mel)	½ cup	53
(Estee)	½ cup	106
Vanilla:		
(Dia-Mel)	½ cup	50
(D-Zerta)	½ cup	71
(Featherweight) artifically sweetened	½ cup	60
PUDDING STIX (Good Humor)	1¾-fl.-oz. pop	90
PUDDING SUNDAE (Swiss Miss):		
Caramel or mint	4-oz. container	170
Chocolate	4-oz. container	190
Peanut butter	4-oz. container	200
PUFFED RICE:		
(Malt-O-Meal)	1 cup	50
(Quaker)	1 cup	55
PUFFED WHEAT:		
(Malt-O-Meal)	1 cup	50
(Quaker)	1 cup	54
PUMPKIN, canned (Libby's) solid pack	½ cup	80
PUMPKIN SEED, in hull	1 oz.	116

Q

Food and Description	Measure or Quantity	Calories
QUAIL, raw, meat & skin	4 oz.	195
QUIK, (Nestlé) chocolate or strawberry	1 tsp.	45
QUISP, cereal	1⅙ cup	121

R

Food and Description	Measure or Quantity	Calories
RADISH	2 small radishes	4
RAISIN, dried:		
(Del Monte) golden	3 oz.	260
(Sun-Maid)	1 oz.	290
RAISINS, RICE & RYE, cereal		
(Kellogg's)	¾ cup	140
RALSTON, cereal	¼ cup	90
RASPBERRY:		
Fresh:		
Black, trimmed	½ cup	49
Red, trimmed	½ cup	41
Frozen (Birds Eye) quick thaw	5-oz. serving	155
RASPBERRY PRESERVE OR JAM:		
Sweetened (Smucker's)	1 T.	53
Dietetic:		
(Estee, Louis Sherry)	1 T.	6
(Featherweight) red	1 T.	16
(S&W) *Nutradiet,* red	1 T.	12
RATATOUILLE, frozen (Stouffer's)	5-oz. serving	60
RAVIOLI:		
Canned, regular pack		
(Franco-American) beef, *RavioliOs*	7½-oz. serving	210
Canned, dietetic (Estee) beef	8-oz. can	210
Frozen:		
(Buitoni):		
Cheese:		
Regular, square	4.8 oz.	331
Ravioletti	2.6 oz.	221
Meat, square	4.8 oz.	318
(Celantano):		
Regular	6½ oz.	410
Mini	4 oz.	250
(Weight Watchers) baked	8¹⁄₁₆ oz. meal	290
RED LOBSTER RESTAURANTS		
("Lunch portion" refers to a cooked serving weighing 5 oz. raw, unless otherwise noted):		
Calamari, breaded & fried	1 lunch portion	360

129

Food and Description	Measure or Quantity	Calories
Catfish	1 lunch portion	170
Chicken breast	4-oz. serving	120
Clam, cherrystone	1 lunch portion	130
Cod, Atlantic	1 lunch portion	100
Crab legs, king	16 oz.	170
Grouper	1 lunch portion	110
Hamburger, without bun	5.3 oz.	320
Lobster, rock	1 tail	230
Monkfish	1 lunch portion	110
Mussels	3 oz.	70
Oysters	6 raw oysters	110
Pollock	1 lunch portion	120
Salmon, sockeye	1 lunch portion	160
Scallop, deep sea	1 lunch portion	130
Shark, mako	1 lunch portion	140
Shrimp	8-12 pieces	120
Sole, lemon	1 lunch portion	120
Steak:		
Porterhouse	18-oz. serving	1420
Sirloin	7-oz. serving	570
Strip	7-oz. serving	690
Swordfish	1 lunch portion	100
RELISH:		
Dill (Vlasic)	1 oz.	2
Hamburger:		
(Heinz)	1 oz.	30
(Vlasic)	1 T.	24
Hot dog:		
(Heinz)	1 oz.	35
(Vlasic)	1 T.	28
Sweet (Vlasic)	1 T.	18
RENNET MIX (Junket):		
*Powder, any flavor:		
Made with skim milk	½ cup	90
Made with whole milk	½ cup	120
Tablet	1 tablet	1
RHINE WINE:		
(Great Western)	3 fl. oz.	73
(Taylor)	3 fl. oz.	75
RHUBARB, cooked, sweetened	½ cup	169
*RICE:		
Brown (Uncle Ben's) parboiled, with added butter	⅔ cup	152
White:		
(Minute Rice) instant, no added butter	⅔ cup	120
(Success) long grain	½ cooking bag	110
White & wild (Carolina)	½ cup	90
RICE CAKE (Pritikin)	1 cake	35

Food and Description	Measure or Quantity	Calories
RICE, FRIED (See also RICE MIX):		
*Canned (La Choy)	⅓ of 11-oz. can	190
Frozen:		
(Birds Eye)	3.7-oz. serving	104
(Green Giant) *Boil 'N Bag*	10-oz. entree	300
(La Choy) & meat	8-oz. serving	280
RICE, FRIED, SEASONING MIX		
(Kikkoman)	1-oz. pkg.	91
RICE KRINKLES, cereal (Post)	⅞ cup	109
RICE KRISPIES, cereal (Kellogg's):		
Regular, frosted, cocoa or strawberry	1 oz.	110
Marshmallow	1 oz.	140
RICE MIX:		
Beef:		
*(Carolina) *Bake-It-Easy*	¼ pkg.	110
(Lipton) & sauce	¼ pkg.	124
*(Minute Rice)	½ cup	149
Rice-A-Roni	⅙ pkg.	130
Chicken:		
*(Carolina) *Bake-It-Easy*	¼ pkg.	110
(Lipton) & sauce	¼ pkg.	126
Rice-A-Roni	⅙ pkg.	130
*Fried (Minute Rice)	½ cup	160
Herb & butter (Lipton)	¼ pkg.	126
*Long grain & wild (Minute Rice)	½ cup	150
Mushroom (Lipton) & sauce	¼ pkg.	123
*Oriental (Carolina) *Bake-It-Easy*	½ pkg.	120
Spanish:		
*(Carolina) *Bake-It-Easy*	¼ pkg.	110
Rice-A-Roni	⅐ pkg.	110
***RICE SEASONING** (French's)*		
Spice Your Rice:		
Beef flavor & onion or		
cheese & chives	½ cup	160
Buttery herb	½ cup	170
RICE, SPANISH:		
canned:		
Regular pack (Comstock;		
Menner's)	½ of 7½-oz. can	140
Dietetic (Featherweight)		
low sodium	7½-oz. serving	140
Frozen (Birds Eye)	3.7-oz. serving	122
RICE & VEGETABLE, frozen:		
(Birds Eye):		
French style	3.7-oz. serving	117
Peas with mushrooms	2⅓ oz.	109
(Green Giant) *Rice Originals*		
& broccoli in cheese sauce	½ cup	140
Pilaf	½ cup	120

131

Food and Description	Measure or Quantity	Calories
RICE WINE:		
Chinese, 20.7% alcohol	1 fl. oz.	38
Japanese, 10.6% alcohol	1 fl. oz.	72
ROCK & RYE (Mr. Boston)	1 fl. oz.	75
ROE, baked or broiled, cod & shad	4 oz.	143
ROLL OR BUN:		
Commercial type, non-frozen:		
Biscuit (Wonder)	1¼-oz. piece	80
Brown & serve (Wonder)		
Gem Style	1-oz. piece	80
Club (Pepperidge Farm)	1.3-oz. piece	100
Crescent (Pepperidge Farm)		
butter	1-oz. piece	110
Croissant (Pepperidge Farm):		
Butter, cinnamon or		
honey-sesame	2-oz. piece	200
Chocolate	2.4-oz. piece	260
Walnut	2-oz. piece	210
Dinner:		
Home Pride	1-oz. piece	85
(Pepperidge Farm)	.7-oz. piece	60
Finger (Pepperidge Farm) sesame		
or poppy seed	.6-oz. piece	60
Frankfurter:		
(Arnold) Hot Dog	1.3-oz. piece	100
(Pepperidge Farm)	1¾-oz. piece	110
(Wonder)	1-oz. piece	80
French:		
(Arnold) *Francisco,* sourdough	1.1-oz. piece	90
(Pepperidge Farm):		
Small	1.3-oz. piece	110
Large	3-oz. piece	240
Golden Twist (Pepperidge Farm)	1-oz. piece	110
Hamburger:		
(Arnold)	1.4-oz. piece	110
(Pepperidge Farm)	1.5-oz. piece	130
Roman Meal	1.8-oz. piece	193
Hoagie (Wonder)	5-oz. piece	400
Old fashioned (Pepperidge Farm)	.6-oz. piece	60
Parkerhouse (Pepperidge Farm)	.6-oz. piece	50
Party (Pepperidge Farm)	.4-oz. piece	30
Sandwich (Arnold) soft	1.3-oz. piece	110
Soft (Pepperidge Farm)	1¼-oz. piece	110
Frozen:		
Apple crunch (Sara Lee)	1-oz. piece	102
Caramel pecan (Sara Lee)	1.3-oz. piece	161
Cinnamon (Sara Lee)	.9-oz. piece	100
Croissant (Sara Lee)	.9-oz. piece	109
Crumb (Sara Lee) French	1¾-oz. piece	188

Food and Description	Measure or Quantity	Calories
Danish (Sara Lee):		
Apple	1.3-oz. piece	120
Cheese	1.3-oz. piece	130
Cinnamon raisin	1.3-oz. piece	147
Pecan	1.3-oz. piece	148
Honey (Morton) mini	1.3-oz. piece	133
*ROLL OR BUN DOUGH:		
Frozen (Rich's):		
Cinnamon	2¼-oz. piece	173
Frankfurter	1 piece	136
Hamburger, regular	1 piece	134
Parkerhouse	1 piece	82
Refrigerated (Pillsbury):		
Apple danish,	1 piece	240
Caramel danish, with nuts	1 piece	155
Cinnamon raisin danish	1 piece	145
Crescent	1 piece	100
*ROLL MIX, HOT (Pillsbury)	1 piece	120
ROMAN MEAL CEREAL	⅓ cup	103
ROSEMARY LEAVES (French's)	1 tsp.	5
ROSÉ WINE:		
Corbett Canyon (Glenmore)	3 fl. oz.	63
(Great Western)	3 fl. oz.	80
(Paul Masson):		
Regular, 11.8% alcohol	3 fl. oz.	76
Light, 7.1% alcohol	3 fl. oz.	49
ROY ROGERS:		
Bar Burger, R.R.	1 burger	611
Biscuit	1 biscuit	231
Breakfast crescent sandwich:		
Regular	4.5-oz. sandwich	401
With bacon	4.7-oz. sandwich	431
With ham	5.8-oz. sandwich	557
With sausage	5.7-oz. sandwich	449
Brownie	1 piece	264
Cheeseburger:		
Regular	1 burger	563
With bacon	1 burger	581
Chicken:		
Breast	1 piece	412
Leg	1 piece	140
Thigh	1 piece	296
Wing	1 piece	192
Coleslaw	3½-oz. serving	110
Danish:		
Apple	1 piece	249
Cheese	1 piece	254
Cherry	1 piece	271

Food and Description	Measure or Quantity	Calories
Drinks:		
Coffee, black	6 fl. oz.	Tr.
Coke:		
Regular	12 fl. oz.	145
Diet	12 fl. oz.	1
Hot chocolate	6 fl. oz.	123
Milk	8 fl. oz.	150
Orange juice:		
Regular	7 fl. oz.	99
Large	10 fl. oz.	136
Shake:		
Chocolate	1 shake	358
Strawberry	1 shake	306
Vanilla	1 shake	315
Tea, iced, plain	8 fl. oz.	0
Egg & biscuit platter:		
Regular	1 meal	394
With bacon	1 meal	435
With ham	1 meal	442
With sausage	1 meal	550
Hamburger	1 burger	456
Pancake platter, with syrup & butter		
Plain	1 order	452
With bacon	1 order	493
With ham	1 order	506
With sausage	1 order	608
Potato:		
Baked, *Hot Topped:*		
Plain	1 potato	211
With bacon & cheese	1 potato	397
With broccoli & cheese	1 potato	376
With margarine	1 potato	274
With sour cream & chives	1 potato	408
With taco beef & cheese	1 potato	463
French fries:		
Regular	3 oz.	268
Large	4 oz.	357
Potato salad	3½-oz. order	107
Roast beef sandwich:		
Plain:		
Regular	1 sandwich	317
Large	1 sandwich	360
With cheese:		
Regular	1 sandwich	424
Large	1 sandwich	467
Salad bar:		
Bacon bits	1 T.	33
Beets, sliced	¼ cup	16
Broccoli	½ cup	20

Food and Description	Measure or Quantity	Calories
Carrot, shredded	¼ cup	42
Cheese, cheddar	¼ cup	112
Croutons	1 T.	35
Egg, chopped	1 T.	27
Lettuce	1 cup	10
Macaroni salad	1 T.	30
Mushrooms	¼ cup	5
Noodle, Chinese	¼ cup	55
Pepper, green	1 T.	2
Potato salad	1 T.	25
Tomato	1 slice	7
Salad dressing:		
Regular:		
Bacon & tomato	1 T.	68
Bleu cheese	1 T.	75
Ranch	1 T.	77
1,000 Island	1 T.	80
Low calorie, Italian	1 T.	35
Strawberry shortcake	7.2-oz. serving	447
Sundae:		
Caramel	1 sundae	293
Hot fudge	1 sundae	337
Strawberry	1 sundae	216
RUTABAGA:		
Canned (Sunshine) solids & liq.	½ cup	32
Frozen (Sunshine)	4 oz.	50

S

Food and Description	Measure or Quantity	Calories
SAFFLOWER SEED, in hull	1 oz.	89
SAGE (French's)	1 tsp.	4
SAKE WINE	1 fl. oz.	39
SALAD CRUNCHIES (Libby's)	1 T.	35
SALAD DRESSING:		
Regular:		
Bacon (Seven Seas) creamy	1 T.	60
Bacon & tomato (Henri's)	1 T.	70
Bleu or blue cheese		
(Wish-Bone) chunk	1 T.	70
Caesar:		
(Pfeiffer)	1 T.	70
(Seven Seas) *Viva*	1 T.	60
Capri (Seven Seas)	1 T.	70
Cheddar & bacon (Wish-Bone)	1 T.	70
Cucumber (Wish-Bone)	1 T.	80
French:		
(Bernstein's) creamy	1 T.	56
(Henri's):		
Hearty	1 T.	70
Original	1 T.	60
(Seven Seas) creamy	1 T.	60
(Wish-Bone) garlic or herbal	1 T.	60
Garlic (Wish-Bone) creamy	1 T.	74
Green Goddess (Seven Seas)	1 T.	60
Herb & spice (Seven Seas)	1 T.	60
Italian:		
(Bernstein's)	1 T.	50
(Henri's):		
Authentic	1 T.	80
Creamy garlic	1 T.	50
(Pfeiffer) chef	1 T.	60
(Seven Seas) *Viva!*	1 T.	70
(Wish-Bone) regular or herbal	1 T.	70
Miracle Whip (Kraft)	1 T.	70
Ranchouse (Henri's) *Chef's Recipe*	1 T.	70
Red wine vinegar & oil		
(Seven Seas)	1 T.	60

Food and Description	Measure or Quantity	Calories
Roquefort:		
(Bernstein's)	1 T.	65
(Marie's)	1 T.	105
Russian:		
(Henri's)	1 T.	60
(Pfeiffer)	1 T.	65
(Wish-Bone)	1 T.	47
Sour cream & bacon (Wish-Bone)	1 T.	70
Spin Blend (Hellmann's)	1 T.	57
Thousand Island:		
(Pfeiffer)	1 T.	65
(Wish-Bone) plain	1 T.	69
Vinaigrette (Bernstein's) French	1 T.	49
Dietetic or low calorie:		
Bacon & tomato (Estee)	1 T.	8
Bleu or blue cheese:		
(Estee)	1 T.	8
(Featherweight) imitation	1 T.	4
(Herni's)	1 T.	30
(Tillie Lewis) *Tasti-Diet*	1 T.	12
(Walden Farms) chunky	1 T.	27
(Wish-Bone) chunky	1 T.	38
Buttermilk (Wish-Bone)	1 T.	53
Caesar:		
(Estee) garlic	1 T.	4
(Featherweight) creamy	1 T.	14
Catalina (Kraft)	1 T.	16
Chef's Recipe Ranchouse (Henri's)	1 T.	30
Cucumber (Kraft)	1 T.	30
French:		
(Estee)	1 T.	4
(Featherweight) low calorie	1 T.	6
(Henri's) original	1 T.	40
(Pritikin)	1 T.	10
(Walden Farms)	1 T.	33
(Wish-Bone)	1 T.	31
Herb & spice (Featherweight)	1 T.	6
Garlic (Estee)	1 T.	2
Italian:		
(Estee) creamy	1 T.	6
(Henri's) creamy	1 T.	25
(Pritikin) creamy	1 T.	16
(Walden Farms)	1 T.	9
(Weight Watchers)	1 T.	50
(Wish-Bone)	1 T.	30
Onion & chive (Wish-Bone)	1 T.	40
Onion & cucumber (Estee)	1 T.	6
Ranch (Pritikin)	1 T.	18
Red wine/vinegar (Featherweight)	1 T.	6

Food and Description	Measure or Quantity	Calories
Russian:		
(Featherweight) creamy	1 T.	6
(Pritikin)	1 T.	12
(Weight Watchers)	1 T.	50
(Wish-Bone)	1 T.	22
Tas-Tee (Henri's)	1 T.	30
Thousand Island:		
(Estee)	1 T.	6
(Henri's)	1 T.	30
(Kraft)	1 T.	30
(Walden Farms)	1 T.	24
(Weight Watchers)	1 T.	50
(Wish-Bone)	1 T.	40
Tomato (Pritikin) zesty	1 T.	18
2-Calorie Low Sodium		
(Featherweight)	1 T.	2
Whipped (Tillie Lewis) *Tasti Diet*	1 T.	18
Yoganaise (Henri's)	1 T.	60
SALAD DRESSING MIX:		
*Regular (Good Seasons):		
Blue cheese & herbs	1 T.	80
Buttermilk, farm style	1 T.	60
Garlic, cheese	1 T.	80
Garlic & herb	1 T.	80
Italian, regular, cheese or zesty	1 T.	80
Dietetic:		
*Blue cheese (Weight Watchers)	1 T.	10
*French (Weight Watchers)	1 T.	4
Garlic (Dia-Mel)	½-oz. pkg.	21
*Italian:		
(Good Seasons) regular	1 T.	25
(Weight Watchers):		
Regular	1 T.	2
Creamy	1 T.	4
*Russian (Weight Watchers)	1 T.	4
*Thousand Island		
(Weight Watchers)	1 T.	12
SALAD SUPREME (McCormick)	1 tsp.	11
SALAMI:		
(Eckrich) for beer or cooked	1 oz.	70
(Hormel):		
Beef	1 slice	40
Genoa, DiLusso	1-oz. serving	100
Hard, sliced	1 slice	34
(Ohse) cooked	1 oz.	65
(Oscar Mayer):		
For beer, beef	.8-oz. slice	66
Cotto	.8-oz. slice	54
Genoa	.3-oz. slice	35

138

Food and Description	Measure or Quantity	Calories
SALISBURY STEAK, frozen:		
(Armour) *Classic Lite*	10-oz. meal	290
(Banquet):		
Buffet Supper	2-lb. pkg.	1260
Man Pleaser	19-oz. dinner	1024
(Stouffer's) *Lean Cuisine*	9½-oz. pkg.	270
(Swanson):		
Regular:		
Dinner, 4-compartment	11-oz. dinner	460
Entree	5½-oz. entree	370
Hungry Man	16½-oz. dinner	710
Main Course	8½-oz. entree	430
(Weight Watchers) beef, Romano	8¾-oz. meal	300
SALMON:		
Baked or broiled	6¾" × 2½" × 1" piece	264
Canned, regular pack, solids & liq.:		
Keta (Bumble Bee)	½ cup	153
Pink or Humpback:		
(Bumble Bee)	½ cup	155
(Del Monte)	7¾-oz. can	290
Sockeye or Red or Blueback:		
(Bumble Bee)	½ cup	188
(Libby's)	7¾-oz. can	380
Canned, dietetic (S&W) *Nutradiet*, low sodium	½ cup	188
SALMON, SMOKED (Vita):		
Lox, drained	4-oz. jar	136
Nova, drained	4-oz. can	221
SALT:		
(Morton):		
Regular	1 tsp.	0
Lite	1 tsp.	0
Substitute:		
(Adolph's) plain	1 tsp.	1
(Morton) plain	1 tsp.	Tr.
Salt-It (Estee)	1 tsp.	0
SALT 'N SPICE SEASONING (McCormick)	1 tsp.	3
SANDWICH SPREAD:		
(Hellmann's)	1 T.	65
(Oscar Mayer)	1-oz. serving	67
SANGRIA (Taylor)	3 fl. oz.	99
SARDINE, canned:		
Atlantic (Del Monte) with tomato sauce	7½-oz. can	319
Imported (Underwood) in mustard or tomato sauce	3¾-oz. can	220
Norwegian:		
(Granadaisa Brand) in tomato sauce	3¾-oz. can	195

Food and Description	Measure or Quantity	Calories
(King David Brand) brisling in olive oil	3¾-oz. can	293
(Queen Helga Brand) in sild oil	3¾-oz. can	310
SAUCE:		
Regular:		
A-1	1 T.	12
Barbecue:		
Chris & Pitt's	1 T.	15
(Gold's)	1 T.	25
(Heinz)	¼ cup	80
(Hunt's) hickory or hot & zesty	1 T.	25
(Kraft) plain or hot	¼ cup	80
Open Pit (General Foods) original, hot n' spicy or smoke flavor	1 T.	25
Burrito (Del Monte)	¼ cup	20
Cheese (Snow's) welsh rarebit	½ cup	170
Chili (See CHILI SAUCE)		
Cocktail:		
(Gold's)	1 T.	31
(Pfeiffer)	1-oz. serving	100
Escoffier Sauce Diable	1 T.	20
Escoffier Sauce Robert	1 T.	20
Famous Sauce	1 T.	69
Hot, (Gebhardt)	1 tsp.	0
Italian (See also SPAGHETTI SAUCE or TOMATO SAUCE):		
(Contadina)	4-oz. serving	71
(Ragú) red cooking	3½-oz. serving	45
Newberg (Snow's)	⅓ cup	120
Salsa Mexicana (Contadina)	4 fl. oz.	38
Salsa Picante (Del Monte) regular	¼ cup	20
Salsa Roja (Del Monte)	¼ cup	20
Seafood cocktail (Del Monte)	1 T.	21
Soy:		
(Chun King)	1 T.	5
(Gold's)	1 T.	10
(Kikkoman) light	1 T.	9
(La Choy)	1 T.	8
Spare rib (Gold's)	1 T.	51
Steak (Dawn Fresh) with mushrooms	1-oz. serving	9
Steak Supreme	1 T.	20
Sweet & sour:		
(Chun King)	1.8 oz.	57
(Contadina)	4 fl. oz.	150
(La Choy)	1-oz. serving	43
Swiss steak (Carnation)	2-oz. serving	20
Tabasco	¼ tsp.	Tr.

Food and Description	Measure or Quantity	Calories
Taco:		
Old El Paso, hot or mild	1 T.	5
(Ortega) hot or mild	1 oz.	13
Tartar:		
(Hellmann's)	1 T.	73
(Nalley's)	1 T.	89
Teriyaki (Kikkoman)	1 T.	12
V-8	1-oz. serving	25
White, medium	¼ cup	103
Worcestershire:		
(French's) regular or smoky	1 T.	10
(Gold's)	1 T.	42
Dietetic (Estee):		
Barbecue	1 T.	16
Cocktail	1 T.	10
Taco	1 oz.	14
SAUCE MIX:		
Regular:		
A la King (Durkee)	1-oz. pkg.	133
*Cheese:		
(Durkee)	½ cup	168
(French's)	½ cup	160
Hollandaise:		
(Durkee)	1-oz. pkg.	173
*(French's)	1 T.	15
*Sour cream (French's)	2½ T.	60
*Sweet & sour (Kikkoman)	1 T.	18
Teriyaki (Kikkoman)	1.5-oz. pkg.	125
*White (Durkee)	1 cup	238
*Dietetic (Weight Watchers) lemon butter	1 T.	8
SAUERKRAUT, canned:		
(Claussen) drained	½ cup	16
(Comstock) regular	½ cup	30
(Del Monte) solids & liq.	1 cup	55
(Silver Floss) solids & liq.:		
Regular	½ cup	30
Krispy Kraut	½ cup	25
(Vlasic)	2 oz.	8
SAUSAGE:		
*Brown & Serve (Hormel)	1 sausage	70
Links (Ohse) hot	1 oz.	80
Patty (Hormel)	1 patty	150
Polish-style:		
(Eckrich)	1-oz. serving	95
(Hormel) *Kilbase*	1-oz. serving	122
(Ohse) regular	1 oz.	80
Pork:		
(Eckrich)	1-oz. link	100

Food and Description	Measure or Quantity	Calories
*(Hormel) *Little Sizzlers*	1 link	51
(Jimmy Dean)	2-oz. serving	227
*(Oscar Mayer) *Little Friers*	1 link	82
Roll (Eckrich) minced	1-oz. slice	80
Smoked:		
(Eckrich) beef, *Smok-Y-Links*	.8-oz. link	70
(Hormel) smokies	1 sausage	80
(Ohse)	1 oz.	80
(Oscar Mayer) beef	1½-oz. link	123
*Turkey (Louis Rich) links or tube	1-oz. serving	45
Vienna:		
(Hormel) regular	1 sausage	50
(Libby's) in barbecue sauce	2½-oz. serving	180
SAUTERNE:		
(Great Western)	3 fl. oz.	79
(Taylor)	3 fl. oz.	81
SCALLOP:		
Steamed	4-oz. serving	127
Frozen:		
(Mrs. Paul's) breaded & fried	3½-oz. serving	210
(Stouffer's) *Lean Cuisine*	11-oz. pkg.	230
SCHNAPPS, APPLE (Mr. Boston)	1 fl. oz.	78
SCHNAPPS, PEPPERMINT		
(Mr. Boston)	1 fl. oz.	115
SCREWDRIVER COCKTAIL		
(Mr. Boston) 12½% alcohol	3 fl. oz.	111
SCROD DINNER OR ENTREE,		
frozen (Gorton's) *Light Recipe*	1 pkg.	260
SEAFOOD NEWBERG, frozen:		
(Armour) *Dinner Classics*	10½-oz. meal	280
(Mrs. Paul's)	8½ oz.	310
SEAFOOD PLATTER, frozen		
(Mrs. Paul's) breaded & fried	9-oz. serving	510
SEGO DIET FOOD, canned:		
Regular	10-fl.-oz. can	225
Lite	10-fl.-oz. can	150
SELTZER (Canada Dry)	Any quantity	0
SERUTAN	1 tsp.	6
SESAME SEEDS (French's)	1 tsp.	9
7-GRAIN CEREAL		
(Loma Linda)	1 oz.	110
SHAD, CREOLE	4-oz. serving	172
SHAKE 'N BAKE:		
Chicken, original	1 pkg.	320
Fish	2-oz. pkg.	280
Italian	1 pkg.	320
Pork, barbecue	1 pkg.	320
SHAKEY'S		
Chicken, fried, & potatoes:		
3-piece	1 order	947

Food and Description	Measure or Quantity	Calories
5-piece	1 order	1700
Ham & cheese sandwich	1 sandwich	550
Pizza:		
Cheese:		
Thin	13″ pizza	1403
Thick	13″ pizza	1890
Onion, green pepper, olive & mushroom:		
Thin	13″ pizza	1713
Thick	13″ pizza	2200
Pepperoni:		
Thin	13″ pizza	1833
Thick	13″ pizza	2320
Sausage & mushroom:		
Thin	13″ pizza	1759
Thick	13″ pizza	2256
Sausage & pepperoni:		
Thin	13″ pizza	2111
Thick	13″ pizza	2598
Special:		
Thin	13″ pizza	2110
Thick	13″ pizza	2597
Potatoes	15-piece order	950
Spaghetti with meat sauce & garlic bread	1 order	940
Super hot hero	1 sandwich	810
SHELLS, PASTA, STUFFED, frozen:		
(Celentano):		
Broccoli & cheese	11½-oz. pkg.	400
Cheese:		
Without sauce	½ of 12½-oz. pkg.	350
With sauce	½ of 16-oz. pkg.	320
(Stouffer's) cheese stuffed	9-oz. serving	320
***SHELLS AND SAUCE** (Lipton):		
Creamy garlic	½ cup	144
Herb tomato	½ cup	130
SHERBET OR SORBET:		
Cassis (Häagen-Dazs)	4 fl. oz.	128
Daiquiri Ice (Häagen-Dazs)	4 fl. oz.	136
Lemon (Häagen-Dazs)	4 fl. oz.	140
Orange:		
(Baskin-Robbins)	4 fl. oz.	158
(Häagen-Dazs)	4 fl. oz.	140
SHERRY:		
Cocktail (Gold Seal)	3 fl. oz.	122
Cream (Great Western) Solera	3 fl. oz.	141
Dry (Williams & Humbert)	3 fl. oz.	120
Dry Sack (Williams & Humbert)	3 fl. oz.	120

Food and Description	Measure or Quantity	Calories
SHREDDED WHEAT:		
(Nabisco):		
Regular size	¾-oz. biscuit	90
Spoon Size	⅔ cup	110
(Quaker)	1 biscuit	52
(Sunshine):		
Regular	1 biscuit	90
Bite size	⅔ cup	110
SHRIMP:		
Canned (Bumble Bee) solids & liq.	4½-oz. can	90
Frozen (Mrs. Paul's):		
Breaded & fried	3 oz.	190
Parmesan	11-oz. meal	310
SHRIMP COCKTAIL canned or		
frozen (Sau-Sea)	4 oz.	113
SHRIMP DINNER, frozen:		
(Armour) *Classic Lites,* in sherried		
cream sauce	10½-oz. meal	280
(Blue Star) *Dining Lite,* creole	10-oz. meal	210
(Conagra) *Light & Elegant*	10-oz. meal	218
(Stouffer's) Newberg	6½-oz. serving	300
SLENDER (Carnation):		
Bar	1 bar	135
Dry	1 packet	110
Liquid	10-fl.-oz. can	220
SLOPPY HOT DOG SEASONING		
MIX (French's)	1½-oz. pkg.	160
SLOPPY JOE:		
Canned:		
(Hormel) *Short Orders*	7½-oz. can	340
(Libby's):		
Beef	⅓ cup	110
Pork	⅓ cup	120
Frozen (Banquet) *Cookin' Bag*	5-oz. pkg.	199
SLOPPY JOE SAUCE		
(Ragú) *Joe Sauce*	3½ oz.	50
SLOPPY JOE SEASONING MIX:		
*(Durkee) pizza flavor	1¼ cups	746
(French's)	1 pkg.	128
SMURF BERRY CRUNCH, cereal		
(Post)	1 cup	116
SNACK BAR (Pepperidge Farm):		
Apple nut, apricot-raspberry		
or blueberry	1.7-oz. piece	170
Brownie nut or date nut	1½-oz. piece	190
Chocolate chip or coconut macaroon	1½-oz. piece	210
SNO BALL (Hostess)	1 piece	149
SOAVE WINE (Antinori)	3 fl. oz.	84

144

Food and Description	Measure or Quantity	Calories
SOFT DRINK:		
Sweetened:		
Apple (Slice)	6 fl. oz.	98
Birch beer (Canada Dry)	6 fl. oz.	82
Bitter lemon:		
(Canada Dry)	6 fl. oz.	75
(Schweppes)	6 fl. oz.	82
Bubble Up	6 fl. oz.	73
Cactus Cooler (Canada Dry)	6 fl. oz.	90
Cherry:		
(Canada Dry) wild	6 fl. oz.	98
(Shasta) black	6 fl. oz.	81
Cherry-lime (Spree)	6 fl. oz.	79
Chocolate (Yoo-Hoo)	6 fl. oz.	93
Club	Any quantity	0
Cola:		
Coca-Cola:		
Regular or caffeine-free	6 fl. oz.	71
Classic	6 fl. oz.	61
Jamaica (Canada Dry)	6 fl. oz.	79
Pepsi-Cola, regular or		
Pepsi Free	6 fl. oz.	80
(Shasta) regular	6 fl. oz.	72
(Slice)	6 fl. oz.	82
(Spree)	6 fl. oz.	73
Collins mix (Canada Dry)	6 fl. oz.	60
Cream:		
(Canada Dry) vanilla	6 fl. oz.	97
(Schweppes)	6 fl. oz.	86
Dr. Nehi (Royal Crown)	6 fl. oz.	82
Dr Pepper	6 fl. oz.	75
Fruit punch:		
(Nehi)	6 fl. oz.	99
(Shasta)	6 fl. oz.	87
Ginger ale:		
(Canada Dry) regular	6 fl. oz.	68
(Fanta)	6 fl. oz.	60
(Shasta)	6 fl. oz.	60
(Spree)	6 fl. oz.	60
Ginger beer (Schweppes)	6 fl. oz.	70
Grape:		
(Fanta)	6 fl. oz.	81
(Hi-C)	6 fl. oz.	74
(Nehi)	6 fl. oz.	96
(Schweppes)	6 fl. oz.	95
(Welch's) sparkling	6 fl. oz.	90
Grapefruit (Spree)	6 fl. oz.	77
Half & half (Canada Dry)	6 fl. oz.	82
Hi-Spot (Canada Dry)	6 fl. oz.	75

Food and Description	Measure or Quantity	Calories
Lemon lime:		
(Minute Maid)	6 fl.oz.	67
(Shasta)	6 fl. oz.	73
(Spree)	6 fl. oz.	77
Lemon-tangerine (Spree)	6 fl. oz.	82
Mello Yello	6 fl. oz.	81
Mountain Dew	6 fl. oz.	89
Mr. PiBB	6 fl. oz.	68
Orange:		
(Canada Dry) *Sunrise*	6 fl. oz.	97
(Hi-C)	6 fl. oz.	74
(Slice)	6 fl. oz.	97
(Sunkist)	6 fl. oz.	96
Peach (Nehi)	6 fl. oz.	101
Pineapple (Canada Dry)	6 fl. oz.	82
Quinine or tonic water		
(Canada Dry; Schweppes)	6 fl. oz.	68
Root beer:		
Barrelhead (Canada Dry)	6 fl. oz.	82
(Dad's)	6 fl. oz.	83
Rooti (Canada Dry)	6 fl. oz.	79
(Shasta) draft	6 fl. oz.	77
(Spree)	6 fl. oz.	77
7-Up	6 fl. oz.	72
Slice	6 fl. oz.	76
Sprite	6 fl. oz.	68
Strawberry (Shasta)	6 fl. oz.	73
Tahitian Treat (Canada Dry)	6 fl. oz.	97
Tropical blend (Spree)	6 fl. oz.	73
Upper Ten (Royal Crown)	6 fl. oz.	84
Dietetic:		
Apple (Slice)	6 fl. oz.	2
Birch beer (Shasta)	6 fl. oz.	2
Bubble Up	6 fl. oz.	1
Cherry (Shasta) black	6 fl. oz.	0
Chocolate (Shasta)	6 fl. oz.	0
Coffee (No-Cal)	6 fl. oz.	1
Cola:		
(Canada Dry; Shasta)	6 fl. oz.	0
Coca-Cola, regular or caffeine free	6 fl. oz.	<1
Diet Rite	6 fl. oz.	<1
Pepsi, diet, light or caffeine free	6 fl. oz.	<1
(Slice)	6 fl. oz.	10
Cream (Shasta)	6 fl. oz.	<1
Dr Pepper	6 fl. oz.	<2
Fresca	6 fl. oz.	2

Food and Description	Measure or Quantity	Calories
Ginger Ale:		
(Canada Dry)	6 fl. oz.	1
(No-Cal)	6 fl. oz.	0
Grape (Shasta)	6 fl. oz.	0
Grapefruit (Shasta)	6 fl. oz.	2
Lemon-lime (Minute Maid)	6 fl.oz.	9
Mr. PiBB	6 fl. oz.	<1
Orange:		
(Canada Dry; No-Cal)	6 fl. oz.	1
(Minute Maid)	6 fl. oz.	8
(Shasta)	6 fl. oz.	<1
Quinine or tonic (No-Cal)	6 fl. oz.	3
RC 100 (Royal Crown)		
caffeine free	6 fl. oz.	<1
Red Pop (Shasta)	6 fl. oz.	0
Root beer:		
Barrelhead (Canada Dry)	6 fl. oz.	1
(Dad's; Ramblin'; Shasta)	6 fl. oz.	<1
7-Up	6 fl. oz.	2
Slice	6 fl. oz.	13
Sprite	6 fl. oz.	1
Tab, regular or caffeine free	6 fl. oz.	<1
SOLE, frozen:		
(Frionor) *Norway Gourmet*	4-oz. fillet	60
(Mrs. Paul's) fillets,		
breaded & fried	6-oz. serving	280
(Van De Kamp's) batter dipped,		
french fried	1 piece	140
(Weight Watchers) in lemon sauce	9⅛-oz. meal	200
SOUFFLE, frozen (Stouffer's):		
Cheese	6-oz. serving	355
Corn	4-oz. serving	155
SOUP:		
Canned, regular pack:		
*Asparagus (Campbell),		
condensed, cream of:		
Regular	8-oz. serving	90
Creamy Natural	8-oz. serving	200
Bean:		
(Campbell):		
Chunky, with ham,		
old fashioned	11-oz. can	290
*Condensed, with bacon	8-oz. serving	150
(Grandma Brown's)	8-oz. serving	182
Bean, black:		
*(Campbell) condensed	8-oz. serving	110
(Crosse & Blackwell)	6½-oz. serving	80

Food and Description	Measure or Quantity	Calories
Beef:		
(Campbell):		
Chunky:		
Regular	10¾-oz. can	190
Stroganoff	10¾-oz. can	300
*Condensed:		
Regular	8-oz. serving	80
Broth	8-oz. serving	15
Consommé	8-oz. serving	25
Noodle, home style	8-oz. serving	90
(College Inn) broth	1 cup	18
(Swanson) Broth	7¼-oz. can	20
*Broccoli (Campbell) condensed, Creamy Natural	8-oz. serving	140
Celery:		
*(Campbell) condensed, cream of	8-oz. serving	100
*(Rokeach):		
Prepared with milk	10-oz. serving	190
Prepared with water	10-oz. serving	90
*Cheddar cheese (Campbell)	8-oz. serving	130
Chicken:		
(Campbell):		
Chunky:		
& rice	19-oz. can	280
vegetable	19-oz. can	340
*Condensed:		
Alphabet	8-oz. serving	80
Broth:		
Plain	8-oz. serving	35
& rice	8-oz. serving	50
Cream of	8-oz. serving	110
Gumbo	8-oz. serving	60
Mushroom, creamy	8-oz. serving	120
Noodle:		
Regular	8-oz. serving	70
NoodleOs	8-oz. serving	70
& rice	8-oz. serving	60
Vegetable	8-oz. serving	70
*Semi-condensed, Soup For One,		
Vegetable, full flavored	11-oz. serving	120
(College Inn) broth	1 cup	35
(Swanson) broth	7¼-oz. can	30
Chili beef (Campbell) Chunky	11-oz. can	290
Chowder:		
Beef'n vegetable (Hormel) Short Orders	7½-oz. can	120

Food and Description	Measure or Quantity	Calories
Clam:		
Manhattan style:		
(Campbell):		
Chunky	19-oz. can	300
*Condensed	8-oz. serving	70
(Crosse & Blackwell)	6½-oz. serving	50
*(Snow's) condensed	7½-oz. serving	70
New England style:		
*(Campbell):		
Condensed:		
Made with milk	8-oz. serving	150
Made with water	8-oz. serving	80
Semi-condensed,		
Soup for One:		
Made with milk	11-oz. serving	190
Made with water	11-oz. serving	130
(Crosse & Blackwell)	6½-oz. serving	90
*(Gorton's)	1 can	560
*(Snow's) condensed, made		
with milk	7½-oz. serving	140
*Fish (Snow's) condensed,		
made with milk	7½-oz. serving	130
Ham'n potato (Hormel)	7½-oz. can	130
Consommé madrilene		
(Crosse & Blackwell)	6½-oz. serving	25
Crab (Crosse & Blackwell)	6½-oz. serving	50
Gazpacho (Crosse & Blackwell)'	6½-oz. serving	30
Ham'n butter bean (Campbell)		
Chunky	10¾-oz. can	280
Lentil (Crosse & Blackwell)		
with ham	6½-oz. serving	80
*Meatball alphabet (Campbell)		
condensed	8-oz. serving	100
Minestrone:		
(Campbell):		
Chunky	19-oz. can	280
*Condensed	8-oz. serving	80
(Crosse & Blackwell)	6½-oz. serving	90
Mushroom:		
*(Campbell):		
Condensed:		
Cream of	8-oz. serving	100
Golden	8-oz. serving	80
(Crosse & Blackwell) cream of,		
bisque	6½-oz. serving	90
*(Rokeach) cream of:		
Prepared with milk	10-oz. serving	240
Prepared with water	10-oz. serving	150

Food and Description	Measure or Quantity	Calories
*Noodle (Campbell) & ground beef	8-oz. serving	90
*Onion (Campbell):		
Regular	8-oz. serving	60
Cream of:		
Made with water	8-oz. serving	100
Made with water & milk	8-oz. serving	140
*Oyster stew (Campbell):		
Made with milk	8-oz. serving	150
Made with water	8-oz. serving	80
*Pea, green (Campbell)	8-oz. serving	160
Pea, split:		
(Campbell):		
Chunky, with ham	19-oz. can	400
*Condensed, with ham & bacon	8-oz. serving	160
(Grandma Brown's)	8-oz. serving	184
*Pepper pot (Campbell)	8-oz. serving	90
*Potato (Campbell) cream of:		
Regular:		
Made with water	8-oz. serving	70
Made with water & milk	8-oz. serving	110
Creamy Natural	8-oz. serving	220
Shav (Gold's)	8-oz. serving	11
Shrimp:		
*(Campbell) condensed, cream of:		
Made with milk	8-oz. serving	160
Made with water	8-oz. serving	90
(Crosse & Blackwell)	6½-oz. serving	90
*Spinach (Campbell) condensed, *Creamy Natural*	8-oz. serving	160
Steak & potato (Campbell) *Chunky*	19-oz. can	340
Tomato:		
(Campbell):		
Condensed:		
Regular:		
Made with milk	8-oz. serving	160
Made with water	8-oz. serving	90
& rice, old fashioned	8-oz. serving	110
Creamy Natural	8-oz. serving	190
Semi-condensed, *Soup For One*, Royale	11-oz. serving	180
*(Rokeach):		
Made with milk	10-oz. serving	190
Made with water	10-oz. serving	90
Turkey (Campbell) *Chunky*	18¾-oz. can	300

Food and Description	Measure or Quantity	Calories
Vegetable:		
(Campbell):		
Chunky:		
Regular	19-oz. can	260
Beef, old fashioned	19-oz. can	320
*Condensed:		
Regular	8-oz. serving	80
Beef or vegetarian	10-oz. serving	70
*Semi-condensed,		
Soup For One, old world	11-oz. serving	160
*(Rokeach) vegetarian	10-oz. serving	90
Vichyssoise (Crosse & Blackwell)	6½-oz. serving	70
*Won ton (Campbell)	8-oz. serving	40
Canned, dietetic pack:		
Bean (Pritikin) navy	½ of 14¾-oz. can	130
Beef (Campbell) *Chunky,*		
& mushroom, low sodium	10¾-oz. can	210
Chicken:		
(Campbell) low sodium:		
Regular, with noodles	10¾-oz. can	160
Vegetable	10¾-oz. can	240
*(Estee) & vegetable	7½-oz. serving	120
(Pritikin):		
Broth	½ of 13¾-oz. can	14
Vegetable	½ of 14¾-oz. can	70
Chowder (Pritikin):		
Manhattan	½ of 14¾-oz. can	70
New England	½ of 14¾-oz. can	118
Lentil (Pritikin)	½ of 14¾-oz. can	100
*Minestrone (Estee)	7½-oz. serving	160
Mushroom (Campbell) cream of,		
low sodium	10½-oz. can	200
Onion (Campbell) low sodium	10½-oz. can	80
Pea, split (Campbell) low sodium	10¾-oz. can	240
Tomato: (Campbell) low sodium		
with tomato pieces	10½-oz. can	180
Turkey (Pritikin) vegetable	½ of 14¾-oz. can	50
Vegetable (Campbell) *Chunky*		
low sodium	10¾-oz. can	170
Frozen:		
*Barley & mushroom		
(Tabatchnick)	8-oz. serving	92
Bean (Kettle Ready)	8 oz.	492
Bean & barley (Tabatchnick)	8 oz.	63
Beef (Kettle Ready) vegetable	8 oz.	133
Broccoli, cream of:		
(Kettle Ready)	8 oz.	160
(Tabatchnick)	7½ oz.	90
Cheese, cheddar (Kettle Ready)	8 oz.	219

151

Food and Description	Measure or Quantity	Calories
Chicken, cream of (Kettle Ready)	8 oz.	185
Chowder:		
Clam:		
Boston (Kettle Ready)	8 oz.	199
Manhattan:		
(Kettle Ready)	8 oz.	161
(Tabatchnick)	7½ oz.	94
New England:		
(Kettle Ready)	8-oz.	180
(Tabatchnick)	7½ oz.	97
Corn & broccoli (Kettle Ready)	8 oz.	163
Minestrone (Tabatchnick)	8 oz.	147
Onion (Kettle Ready)	8 oz.	86
Pea, split with ham:		
(Kettle Ready)	8-oz.	189
(Stouffer's)	8¼-oz.	190
Potato (Kettle Ready) cream of	8 oz.	162
Spinach cream of:		
(Kettle Ready)	8 oz.	140
(Stouffer's)	8-oz.	230
(Tabatchnick)	7½ oz.	90
Tomato (Kettle Ready) cream of	8 oz.	267
Vegetable:		
(Kettle Ready) hearty	8 oz.	132
(Tabatchnick)	8 oz.	97
*Won Ton (La Choy)	½ of 15-oz. pkg.	50
Mix, regular:		
Beef:		
*Carmel Kosher	6 fl. oz.	12
*(Lipton) Cup-A-Soup:		
Noodle	6 fl. oz.	45
Lots-A-Noodles	7 fl. oz.	120
*(Weight Watchers) broth	6 fl. oz.	10
*Chicken:		
Carmel Kosher	6 fl. oz.	12
(Lipton):		
Cup-A-Broth	6 fl. oz.	25
Cup-A-Soup, & rice	6 fl. oz.	45
Country style, hearty	6 fl. oz.	73
Lots-A-Noodles, regular	7 fl. oz.	120
*Minestrone (Manischewitz)	6 fl. oz.	50
*Mushroom:		
Carmel Kosher	6 fl. oz.	12
(Lipton):		
Regular, beef	8 fl. oz.	40
Cup-A-Soup, cream of	6 fl. oz.	82
*Noodle (Lipton):		
With chicken broth	8 fl. oz.	70
Giggle Noodle	8 fl. oz.	80

Food and Description	Measure or Quantity	Calories
*Onion:		
Carmel Kosher	6 fl. oz.	12
(Lipton):		
Regular, beef	8 fl. oz.	35
Cup-A-Soup	6 fl. oz.	30
*Pea, green (Lipton) *Cup-A-Soup*	6 fl. oz.	115
*Pea, split (Manischewitz)	6 fl. oz.	45
*Tomato (Lipton) *Cup-A-Soup*	6 fl. oz.	100
*Tomato onion (Lipton)	8 fl. oz.	80
*Vegetable:		
(Lipton):		
Regular, country	8 fl. oz.	80
Cup-A-Soup:		
Regular, spring	6 fl. oz.	41
Country style, harvest	6 fl. oz.	94
Lots-A-Noodles, garden	7 fl. oz.	130
(Manischewitz)	6 fl. oz.	50
(Southland) frozen	⅓ of 16-oz. pkg.	60
*Mix, dietetic:		
(Estee):		
Beef noodle	6 fl. oz.	20
Chicken noodle	6 fl. oz.	25
Tomato	6 fl. oz.	40
(Lipton) *Cup-A-Soup-Trim*	6 fl. oz.	10
SOUP GREENS (Durkee)	2⅓-oz. jar	216
SOUTHERN COMFORT:		
80 proof	1 fl. oz.	79
100 proof	1 fl. oz.	95
SOYBEAN CURD OR TOFU	2¾″ × 1½″ × 1″cake	86
SOYBEAN OR NUT:		
Dry roasted (*Soy Ahoy; Soy Town*)	1 oz.	139
Oil roasted (*Soy Ahoy; Soy Town*)		
plain, barbecue or garlic	1 oz.	152
SPAGHETTI:		
Dry (Pritikin) whole wheat	1 oz.	110
Cooked:		
8-10 minutes, "Al Dente"	1 cup	216
14-20 minutes, tender	1 cup	155
Canned:		
(Franco-American):		
In meat sauce	7½-oz. can	210
With meatballs in tomato sauce, *SpaghettiOs*	7⅜-oz. can	210
With sliced franks in tomato sauce, *SpaghettiOs*	7⅜-oz. can	210
(Hormel) *Short Orders,* & meatballs in tomato sauce	7½-oz. can	210
(Libby's) & meatballs in tomato sauce	7½-oz. serving	189

Food and Description	Measure or Quantity	Calories
Dietetic (Estee) & meatballs	7½-oz. serving	240
Frozen:		
(Armour) *Dinner Classics,* with meatballs	11-oz. meal	350
(Banquet) & meat sauce	8-oz. pkg.	270
(Conagra) *Light & Elegant,* & meat sauce	10¼-oz. entree	290
(Morton) & meatball	11-oz. dinner	360
(Stouffer's) *Lean Cuisine*	11½-oz. pkg.	280
(Weight Watchers) with meat sauce	10½-oz. meal	280
SPAGHETTI SAUCE, canned:		
Regular pack:		
Garden Style (Ragú)	4-oz. serving	80
Marinara:		
(Prince)	4-oz. serving	80
(Ragú)	5-oz. serving	120
Meat or meat flavored:		
(Hunt's)	4-oz. serving	70
(Prego)	4-oz. serving	150
(Ragú) regular	4-oz. serving	80
Meatless or plain:		
(Prego)	4-oz. serving	140
(Ragú) regular	4-oz. serving	80
Mushroom:		
(Hain)	4-oz. serving	80
(Hunt's)	4-oz. serving	70
(Prego Plus)	4-oz. serving	130
(Ragú) Extra Thick & Zesty	4-oz. serving	110
Sausage & green pepper (Prego Plus)	4-oz. serving	170
Veal (Prego Plus)	4-oz. serving	150
Dietetic pack:		
(Furman's) low sodium	½ cup	83
(Prego) low sodium	½ cup	100
(Pritikin) plain or mushroom	4-oz. serving	60
*SPAGHETTI SAUCE MIX:		
(Durkee) regular	½ cup	45
(French's) with mushrooms	⅝ cup	100
(Spatini)	½ cup	84
SPAM, luncheon meat (Hormel):		
Regular, smoke flavored or with cheese chunks	1-oz. serving	85
Deviled	1 T.	35
SPARKLING COOLER CITRUS,		
La Croix (Heileman)	6 fl. oz.	107
SPECIAL K, cereal (Kellogg's)	1 cup	110
SPINACH:		
Fresh, whole leaves	½ cup	4

Food and Description	Measure or Quantity	Calories
Boiled	½ cup	18
Canned, regular pack (Allens) solids & liq.	½ cup	25
Canned, dietetic pack (Del Monte) No Salt Added	½ cup	25
Frozen:		
(Birds Eye):		
Chopped or leaf	⅓ pkg.	28
Creamed	⅓ pkg.	60
(Green Giant):		
Creamed	½ cup	70
Harvest Fresh	4-oz. serving	30
(McKenzie) chopped or cut	⅓ pkg.	25
(Stouffer's) souffle	4-oz. serving	135
SPINACH PUREE, canned (Larsen) low sodium	½ cup	22
SQUASH, SUMMER:		
Yellow, boiled slices	½ cup	13
Zucchini, boiled slices	½ cup	9
Canned (Del Monte) zucchini, in tomato sauce	½ cup	30
Frozen:		
(Birds Eye) zucchini	⅓ pkg.	19
(Larsen) yellow crookneck	3.3 oz.	18
(McKenzie) crookneck	⅓ pkg.	20
(Mrs. Paul's) sticks, batter dipped, french fried	⅓ pkg.	180
SQUASH, WINTER:		
Acorn, baked	½ cup	56
Hubbard, baked, mashed	½ cup	51
Frozen:		
(Birds Eye)	⅓ pkg.	43
(Southland) butternut	4-oz. serving	45
STEAK (See BEEF)		
STEAK & GREEN PEPPERS, frozen:		
(Green Giant)	9-oz. entree	250
(Swanson)	8½-oz. entree	200
STEAK UMM	2 oz.	180
STOCK BASE (French's) beef or chicken	1 tsp.	8
STRAWBERRY:		
Fresh, capped	½ cup	26
Frozen (Birds Eye):		
Halves	⅓ pkg.	164
Whole	¼ pkg.	89
Whole, quick thaw	½ pkg.	125
STRAWBERRY DRINK (Hi-C):		
Canned	6 fl. oz.	89
*Mix	6 fl. oz.	68

Food and Description	Measure or Quantity	Calories
STRAWBERRY FRUIT JUICE, canned (Smucker's)	8 fl. oz.	120
STRAWBERRY KRISPIES, cereal (Kellogg's)	¾ cup	110
STRAWBERRY NECTAR, canned (Libby's)	6 fl. oz.	60
STRAWBERRY PRESERVE OR JAM:		
Sweetened:		
(Bama)	1 T.	45
(Smucker's)	1 T.	53
(Welch's)	1 T.	52
Dietetic or low calorie:		
(Estee; Louis Sherry)	1 T.	6
(Diet Delight)	1 T.	12
(Featherweight) calorie reduced	1 T.	16
STUFFING MIX:		
*Beef, *Stove Top*	½ cup	180
*Chicken:		
(Bell's)	½ cup	190
Stove Top	½ cup	180
*Cornbread, *Stove Top*	½ cup	170
Cube or herb seasoned (Pepperidge Farm)	1 oz.	110
*Pork, *Stove Top*	½ cup	170
*Premium Blend (Bell's)	½ cup	180
*Ready Mix (Bell's)	½ cup	224
White bread (Mrs. Cubbison's)	1 oz.	101
STURGEON, smoked	4-oz. serving	169
SUCCOTASH:		
Canned:		
(Comstock) whole kernel	½ cup	80
(Larsen) *Freshlike*	½ cup	80
(Libby's) cream style	½ cup	111
(Stokely-Van Camp)	½ cup	85
Frozen:		
(Birds Eye)	⅓ pkg.	104
(Frosty Acres)	3.3 oz.	100
*SUDDENLY SALADS (General Mills):		
Macaroni, creamy	⅙ of pkg.	200
Pasta, Italian	⅙ of pkg.	160
Potato, creamy	⅙ of pkg.	250
SUGAR:		
Brown	1 T.	48
Confectioners'	1 T.	30
Granulated	1 T.	46
Maple	1¾" × 1¼" × ½" piece	104

Food and Description	Measure or Quantity	Calories
SUGAR CORN POPS, cereal		
(Kellogg's)	1 cup	110
SUGAR CRISP, cereal (Post)	⅞ cup	112
SUGAR PUFFS, cereal		
(Malt-O-Meal)	⅞ cup	110
SUGAR SMACKS, cereal (Kellogg's)	¾ cup	110
SUGAR SUBSTITUTE:		
(Estee)	1 tsp.	12
(Featherweight)	3 drops	0
(Pritikin) *Supreme*	1.76-oz. packet	3
Sprinkle Sweet (Pillsbury)	1 tsp.	2
Sweet'n-it (Estee) liquid	5 drops	0
Sweet 'N Low:		
Brown	1 tsp.	20
Granulated	1-gram packet	4
Liquid	1 drop	0
***SUKIYAKI DINNER** (Chun King)*		
stir fry	6 oz.	257
SUNFLOWER SEED (Fisher):		
In hull, roasted, salted	1 oz.	86
Hulled, dry roasted, salted	1 oz.	164
Hulled, oil roasted, salted	1 oz.	167
SURIMI (See CRAB SUBSTITUTE)		
SUZY Q (Hostess):		
Banana	1 piece	240
Chocolate	1 piece	240
SWEETBREADS, calf, braised	4-oz. serving	191
SWEET POTATO:		
Baked, peeled	5″ × 1″ potato	155
Canned:		
(Allen's)	4-oz. serving	50
(Trappey's) *Sugary Sam:*		
Cut	½ cup (4.3 oz.)	110
Whole	½ cup (4.3 oz.)	130
Frozen:		
(Mrs. Paul's) candied, with apples	4-oz. serving	150
(Stouffer's) & apples	5-oz. serving	160
SWEET & SOUR CHICKEN		
(La Choy):		
*Canned, bi-pack	¾ cup	120
Frozen	12-oz. entree	380
SWISS STEAK, frozen (Swanson)	10-oz. dinner	350
SWORDFISH, broiled	3″ × 3″ × ½″ steak	218
SYRUP (See also TOPPING):		
Regular:		
Apricot (Smucker's)	1 T.	50
Blackberry (Smucker's)	1 T.	50
Chocolate or chocolate-flavored:		
Bosco	1 T.	55

Food and Description	Measure or Quantity	Calories
(Hershey's)	1 T.	40
(Nestlé) *Quik*	1 oz.	80
Corn, *Karo,* dark or light	1 T.	58
Maple, *Karo,* imitation	1 T.	57
Pancake or waffle:		
(Aunt Jemima)	1 T.	53
Golden Griddle	1 T.	54
Karo	1 T.	58
Log Cabin, regular or buttered	1 T.	56
Mrs. Butterworth's	1 T.	55
Strawberry (Smucker's)	1 T.	50
Dietetic or low calorie:		
Blueberry (Estee)	1 T.	4
Chocolate or chocolate-flavored		
(Diet Delight)	1 T.	8
Coffee (No-Cal)	1 T.	6
Cola (No-Cal)	1 T.	0
Maple (S&W) *Nutradiet*	1 T.	12
Pancake or waffle:		
(Aunt Jemima)	1 T.	29
(Cary's)	1 T.	6
(Estee)	1 T.	4
(Featherweight)	1 T.	12

T

Food and Description	Measure or Quantity	Calories
TACO:		
*(Ortega)	1 oz.	54
*Mix (Durkee)	½ cup	321
Shell (Ortega)	1 shell	50
TACO BELL RESTAURANTS:		
Bellbeefer:		
Regular	5-oz. serving	280
With cheese and tomato	5½-oz. serving	305
Burrito:		
Bean	7.2-oz. serving	440
Beef	6.7-oz. serving	430
Combination	8.4-oz. serving	350
Crispas, cinnamon	2.2-oz. serving	230
Enchirato	6.5-oz. serving	325
Nachos:		
Regular	3.3-oz. serving	355
Bellgrande	10.6-oz. serving	725
Pintos and cheese	5.1-oz. serving	225
Taco:		
Regular	3.1-oz. serving	210
Light	5-oz. serving	345
Taco salad	1 serving	910
Tostada, beef	7.4-oz. serving	360
TAMALE:		
Canned:		
(Hormel) beef, *Short Orders*	7½-oz. can	270
Old El Paso, with chili gravy	1 tamale	96
(Pride of Mexico) beef	1 tamale	115
Frozen (Hormel) beef	1 tamale	130
TANG, orange, regular	6 fl. oz.	87
TANGERINE OR		
MANDARIN ORANGE:		
Fresh (Sunkist)	1 large tangerine	39
Canned, solids & liq.:		
Regular pack (Dole)	½ cup	76
Dietetic pack:		
(Diet Delight) juice pack	½ cup	50
(Featherweight) water pack	½ cup	35
(S&W) *Nutradiet*	½ cup	28

Food and Description	Measure or Quantity	Calories
TANGERINE DRINK, canned (Hi-C)	6 fl. oz.	90
TANGERINE JUICE, frozen (Minute Maid)	6 fl. oz.	85
TAPIOCA, dry, *Minute,* quick cooking	1 T.	32
TAQUITO, frozen (Van de Kamp's) beef	8-oz. serving	490
TARRAGON (French's)	1 tsp.	5
TASTEEOS, cereal (Ralston Purina)	1¼ cups	110
TEA:		
Bag:		
(Celestial Seasonings):		
After dinner:		
Amaretto Nights or *Swiss Mint*	1 cup	<3
Bavarian Chocolate Orange	1 cup	7
Caffeine free	1 cup	4
Fruit & tea	1 cup	<3
Herb:		
Almond Sunset, Cinnamon apple or *Cranberry Cove*	1 cup	3
Emperor's Choice or *Lemon Zinger*	1 cup	4
Mandarin Orange Spice or *Orange Zinger*	1 cup	5
Roastaroma	1 cup	11
Premium black tea	1 cup	3
(Lipton):		
Plain or flavored	1 cup	2
Herbal:		
Almond pleasure or cinnamon apple	1 cup	2
Quietly chamomile or toasty spice	1 cup	6
(Sahadi) spearmint	1 cup	4
Instant (Nestea)100%	6 fl. oz.	0
TEAM, cereal	1 cup	110
TEA MIX, ICED:		
*(Lipton) lemon & sugar flavored	1 cup	60
Nestea, lemon-flavored	1 cup	6
*Dietetic, *Crystal Light*	8 fl. oz.	2
TEQUILA SUNRISE COCKTAIL, (Mr. Boston) 12½% alcohol	3 fl. oz.	120
TERIYAKI:		
*Canned (La Choy) chicken	¾ cup	85
Frozen:		
(Armour) *Dinner Classics,* steak	10-oz. meal	360
(Stouffer's) beef	10-oz. serving	365

Food and Description	Measure or Quantity	Calories
TERIYAKI BASTE & GLAZE		
(Kikkoman)	1 T.	28
*TEXTURED VEGETABLE PROTEIN,		
Morningstar Farms:		
Breakfast link	1 link	73
Breakfast patties	1 patty	100
Breakfast strips	1 strip	37
Grillers	1 patty	190
THURINGER:		
(Eckrich) *Smoky Tang*	1-oz. serving	80
(Hormel):		
Beefy	1-oz. serving	100
Old Smokehouse	1-oz. serving	100
(Louis Rich) turkey	1-oz. serving	50
(Ohse) beef	1 oz.	80
(Oscar Mayer)	.8-oz. slice	73
TIGER TAILS (Hostess)	2¼-oz. piece	210
TOASTED WHEAT AND RAISINS,		
cereal (Nabisco)	1 oz.	100
TOASTER CAKE OR PASTRY:		
Pop-Tarts (Kellogg's):		
Regular:		
Blueberry, brown sugar, cinnamon or cherry	1 pastry	210
Strawberry	1 pastry	200
Frosted:		
Blueberry, chocolate fudge or strawberry	1 pastry	200
Brown sugar cinnamon, cherry,	1 pastry	210
Chocolate-vanilla creme	1 pastry	220
Toaster Strudel (Pillsbury)	1 slice	190
Toastettes (Nabisco) regular or frosted	1 piece	200
Toast-R-Cake (Thomas'):		
Blueberry	1 piece	108
Bran	1 piece	103
Corn	1 piece	120
TOASTIES, cereal (Post)	1¼ cups	107
TOASTY O'S, cereal (Malt-O-Meal)	1¼ cup	110
TOFUTTI:		
Frozen:		
Regular:		
Chocolate supreme or wildberry supreme	4 fl. oz.	210
Maple walnut	4 fl. oz.	230
Vanilla	4 fl. oz.	200

Food and Description	Measure or Quantity	Calories
Cuties:		
Chocolate	1 piece	140
Vanilla	1 piece	130
Lite Lite	4 fl. oz.	90
Love Drops:		
Cappuccino or chocolate	4 fl. oz.	230
Vanilla	4 fl. oz.	220
Soft serve:		
Regular	4 fl. oz.	158
Hi-Lite:		
Chocolate	4 fl. oz.	100
Vanilla	4 fl. oz.	90
TOMATO:		
Regular, whole	1 med. tomato	33
Cherry, whole	4 pieces	14
Canned, regular pack, solids & liq.:		
(Contadina) sliced, baby	½ cup	50
(Del Monte) stewed	4 oz.	37
(Hunt's):		
Crushed	½ cup	25
Stewed	½ cup (4 oz.)	35
Whole	4 oz.	20
Canned, dietetic pack, solids & liq.:		
(Del Monte) No Salt Added	½ cup	35
(Featherweight)	½ cup	20
(Furman's) low sodium	½ cup	72
(Hunt's) whole	4 oz.	20
TOMATO & PEPPER, HOT CHILI,		
Old El Paso, Jalapeño	¼ cup	13
TOMATO JUICE, CANNED:		
Regular pack:		
(Campbell; Libby's)	6-fl.-oz. can	35
(Del Monte)	6-fl.-oz. can	36
(Musselman's)	6-fl.-oz. can	30
(Welch's)	6 fl. oz. can	35
Dietetic pack (Diet Delight; Featherweight)	6 fl. oz.	35
TOMATO JUICE COCKTAIL,		
canned:		
(Ocean Spray) *Firehouse Jubilee*	6 fl. oz.	44
SnapE-Tom	6 fl. oz.	40
TOMATO PASTE, canned:		
Regular pack:		
(Contadina) Italian	6-oz. serving	210
(Del Monte)	6-oz. can	150
(Hunt's) Italian style	6 oz.	150
Dietetic (Featherweight) low sodium	6-oz. can	150
TOMATO, PICKLED (Claussen)		
green	1 piece	6

Food and Description	Measure or Quantity	Calories
TOMATO PUREE, canned:		
Regular (Contadina) heavy	1 cup	100
Dietetic (Featherweight)	1 cup	90
TOMATO SAUCE, canned:		
(Contadina) regular	1 cup	90
(Del Monte):		
Regular or No Salt Added	1 cup	70
Hot	½ cup	40
With tomato bits	1 cup	92
(Furman's)	½ cup	58
(Hunt's):		
Regular or with bits	4 oz.	30
With cheese	4 oz.	45
Herbs	4 oz.	80
TOM COLLINS (Mr. Boston) 12½% alcohol	3 fl. oz.	111
***TOM COLLINS MIX,** (Bar-Tender's)	6 fl. oz.	177
TONGUE, beef, braised	4-oz. serving	277
TOPPING:		
Regular:		
Butterscotch (Smucker's)	1 T.	70
Caramel (Smucker's) regular	1 T.	70
Chocolate fudge (Hershey's)	1 T.	50
Nut (Planters)	1 oz.	180
Pecans in syrup (Smucker's)	1 T.	65
Pineapple (Smucker's)	1 T.	65
Strawberry (Smucker's)	1 T.	60
Walnuts in syrup (Smucker's)	1 T.	65
Dietetic, chocolate (Diet Delight)	1 T.	16
TOPPING, WHIPPED:		
Regular:		
Cool Whip (Birds Eye) dairy	1 T.	16
(Johanna) aerosol	1 T.	8
Lucky Whip, aerosol	1 T.	12
Whip Topping (Rich's)	¼ oz.	20
Dietetic (Featherweight)	1 T.	3
*Mix:		
Regular, *Dream Whip*	1 T.	5
Dietetic (D-Zerta; Estee)	1 T.	4
TOP RAMEN, beef (Nissin Foods)	3-oz. serving	390
TORTELLINI, frozen (Buitoni):		
Cheese:		
Regular	2.6 oz.	222
Tricolor	2.6 oz.	221
Meat	2.4 oz.	212
TORTILLA (Amigos)	6″ × ⅛″ tortilla	111
TOSTADA, frozen (Van de Kamp's)	8½-oz. serving	530
TOSTADA SHELL (*Old El Paso*)	1 shell	57

Food and Description	Measure or Quantity	Calories
TOTAL, cereal	1 cup	110
TRIPE, canned (Libby's)	6-oz. serving	290
TRIPLE SEC LIQUEUR		
(Mr. Boston)	1 fl. oz.	79
TRIX, cereal (General Mills)	1 cup	110
TUNA:		
Canned in oil:		
(Bumble Bee):		
Chunk, light, solids & liq.	½ cup	265
Solid, white, solids & liq.	½ cup	285
(Carnation) solids & liq.	6½-oz. can	427
Canned in water:		
(Breast O'Chicken)	6½-oz. can	211
(Bumble Bee):		
Chunk, light, solids & liq.	½ cup	117
Solid, white, solids & liq.	½ cup	126
(Featherweight) light, chunk	6½-oz. can	210
*TUNA HELPER (General Mills):		
Country dumplings or noodles cheese	⅕ pkg.	230
Creamy noodle	⅕ pkg.	280
TUNA PIE, frozen:		
(Banquet)	8-oz. pie	395
(Morton)	8-oz. pie	370
TUNA SALAD:		
Home recipe	4-oz. serving	193
Canned (Carnation)	¼ of 7½-oz. can	100
TURF & SURF DINNER, frozen		
(Armour) *Classic Lights*	10-oz. meal	250
TURKEY:		
Barbecued (Louis Rich) breast, half	1 oz.	40
Packaged:		
(Carl Buddig):		
Regular	1 oz.	50
Ham or salami	1 oz.	40
(Hormel) breast	1 slice	30
(Louis Rich):		
Turkey bologna	1-oz. slice	60
Turkey cotto salami	1-oz. slice	50
Turkey ham, chopped	1-oz. slice	45
Turkey pastrami	1-oz. slice	35
(Ohse):		
Oven cooked	1 oz.	30
Turkey bologna	1 oz.	70
Turkey salami	1 oz.	50
(Oscar Mayer) breast	7½-oz. slice	21
Roasted:		
Flesh & skin	4-oz. serving	253
Dark meat	2½" × 1⅝" × ¼" slice	43
Light meat	4" × 2" × ¼" slice	75

Food and Description	Measure or Quantity	Calories
Smoked (Louis Rich):		
Drumsticks	1 oz. (without bone)	40
Wing drumettes	1 oz. (without bone)	45
TURKEY DINNER OR ENTREE, frozen:		
(Banquet):		
American Favorites	11-oz. dinner	320
Extra Helping	9-oz. dinner	723
(Conagra) *Light & Elegant,* sliced	8-oz. entree	230
(Le Menu) sliced breast, with mushrooms	11¼-oz. dinner	460
(Morton)	11¼-oz. dinner	279
(Swanson):		
Regular	8¾-oz. entree	250
Hungry Man	18½-oz. dinner	590
(Weight Watchers) stuffed, breast	8½-oz. meal	260
TURKEY PIE, frozen:		
(Banquet):		
Regular	8-oz. pie	526
Supreme	8-oz. pie	430
(Morton)	8-oz. pie	340
(Stouffer's)	10-oz. pie	460
(Swanson) chunk	10-oz. pie	530
TURKEY TETRAZZINI, frozen:		
(Stouffer's)	6-oz. serving	240
(Weight Watchers)	10-oz. pkg.	310
TURNIP GREENS, canned (Allen's) chopped, solids & liq.	½ cup	20
TURNIP ROOTS, frozen (McKenzie) diced	1 oz.	4
TURNOVER:		
Frozen (Pepperidge Farm):		
Apple or cherry	1 turnover	310
Blueberry, peach or raspberry	1 turnover	320
Refrigerated (Pillsbury)	1 turnover	170
TWINKIE (Hostess)	1 piece	160

U

Food and Description	Measure or Quantity	Calories
UFO'S, canned (Franco-American):		
Regular	7½ oz.	180
With meteors	7½ oz.	240

V

Food and Description	Measure or Quantity	Calories
VALPOLICELLA WINE (Antinori)	3 fl. oz.	84
VANDERMINT, liqueur	1 fl. oz.	90
VANILLA EXTRACT		
(Virginia Dare)	1 tsp.	10
VEAL, broiled, medium cooked:		
Loin chop	4 oz.	265
Rib, roasted	4 oz.	305
Steak or cutlet, lean & fat	4 oz.	245
VEAL DINNER, frozen:		
(Armour) *Dinner Classics,*		
parmigiana	10¾-oz. meal	400
(Morton) Light	11-oz. dinner	290
(Swanson) parmigiana,		
Hungry Man	20-oz. dinner	640
(Weight Watchers) parmigiana,		
2-compartment	8.625-oz. meal	230
VEAL STEAK, frozen (Hormel):		
Regular	4-oz. serving	130
Breaded	4-oz. serving	240
VEGETABLE BOUILLON		
(Herb-Ox):		
Cube	1 cube	6
Packet	1 packet	12
VEGETABLE JUICE COCKTAIL:		
Regular, *V-8*	6 fl. oz.	35
Dietetic:		
(S&W) *Nutradiet,* low sodium	6 fl. oz.	35
V-8, low sodium	6 fl. oz.	40
VEGETABLES IN PASTRY,		
frozen (Pepperidge Farm):		
Asparagus with mornay sauce or		
broccoli with cheese	3¾ oz.	250
Cauliflower & cheese sauce	3¾ oz.	220
Spinach almondine	3¾ oz.	260
Zucchini provencal	3¾ oz.	210
VEGETABLES, MIXED:		
Canned, regular pack:		
(Del Monte) solids & liq.	½ cup	40

167

Food and Description	Measure or Quantity	Calories
(La Choy):		
Chinese	⅓ of 14-oz. pkg.	12
Chop Suey	½ cup	10
(Libby's) solids & liq.	½ cup	40
(Veg-All)	½ cup	35
Canned, dietetic pack:		
(Featherweight)	½ cup	40
(Larsen) *Fresh-Lite*	½ cup	35
Frozen:		
(Birds Eye):		
Regular:		
Broccoli, cauliflower & carrots in cheese sauce	5 oz.	100
Carrots, peas & onions, deluxe	⅓ pkg.	52
Medley, in butter sauce	⅓ of 10-oz. pkg.	62
Farm Fresh:		
Broccoli, cauliflower & carrot strips	3.2 oz.	25
Brussels sprouts, cauliflower & carrots	3.2 oz.	30
Stir Fry, Chinese style	⅓ pkg.	35
(Chun King) chow mein, drained	4 oz.	32
(Frosty Acres):		
Regular	3.3 oz.	65
Dutch	3.2 oz.	30
Oriental	3.2 oz.	25
Soup mix	3 oz.	45
Stew	3 oz.	42
Swiss mix	3 oz.	25
(Green Giant):		
Regular:		
Broccoli, cauliflower & carrots in cheese sauce	½ cup	60
Corn, broccoli bounty	½ cup	60
Harvest Fresh	½ cup	60
Harvest Get Togethers:		
Broccoli-cauliflower medley	½ cup	60
Broccoli fanfare	½ cup	80
(La Choy) Chinese	4 oz.	25
(Larsen):		
Regular or chuckwagon blend	3.3 oz.	70
California blend or Italian blend	3.3 oz.	30
Oriental blend	3.3 oz.	25
(Southland):		
Gumbo	⅕ of 16-oz. pkg.	40
Stew	4 oz.	60
VEGETABLE STEW, canned *Dinty Moore* (Hormel)	7½-oz. serving	170

Food and Description	Measure or Quantity	Calories
"VEGETARIAN FOODS":		
Canned or dry:		
Chicken, fried (Loma Linda) with gravy	1½-oz. piece	70
Chili (Worthington)	½ cup	177
Choplet (Worthington)	1 choplet	50
Dinner cuts (Loma Linda) drained	1 piece	60
Dinner loaf (Loma Linda)	¼ cup	50
Franks, big (Loma Linda)	1.9-oz. frank	100
Franks, sizzle (Loma Linda)	2.2-oz. frank	85
FriChik (Worthington)	1 piece	75
Little links (Loma Linda) drained	.8-oz. link	40
Non-meatballs (Worthington)	1 meatball	32
Nuteena (Loma Linda)	½" slice	160
Patty mix (Loma Linda)	¼ cup	50
Prime Stakes	1 slice	171
Proteena (Loma Linda)	½" slice	140
Sandwich spread (Loma Linda)	1 T.	23
*Soyagen, all purpose powder (Loma Linda)	1 cup	130
Soyameat (Worthington):		
Beef, sliced	1 slice	44
Chicken, diced	1 oz.	40
Soyameal, any kind (Worthington)	1 oz.	120
Stew pack (Loma Linda) drained	2 oz.	70
Super links (Worthington)	1 link	110
Swiss steak with gravy (Loma Linda)	1 steak	140
Vegelona (Loma Linda)	½" slice	100
Vega-links (Worthington)	1 link	55
Wheat protein	4 oz.	124
Worthington 209	1 slice	58
Frozen:		
Beef pie (Worthington)	1 pie	278
Bologna (Loma Linda)	1 oz.	75
Chicken, fried (Loma Linda)	2-oz. serving	180
Chic-Ketts (Worthington)	1 oz.	53
Corned beef, sliced (Worthington)	1 slice	32
Fri Pats (Worthington)	1 patty	204
Meatballs (Loma Linda)	1 meatball	63
Meatless salami (Worthington)	1 slice	44
Prosage (Worthington)	1 link	60
Smoked beef, slices (Worthington)	1 slice	14
Wham, roll (Worthington)	1 slice	36

Food and Description	Measure or Quantity	Calories
VERMOUTH:		
Dry & extra dry (Lejon; Noilly Pratt)	1 fl. oz.	33
Sweet (Lejon; Taylor)	1 fl. oz.	45
VICHY WATER (Schweppes)	Any quantity	0
VINEGAR	1 T.	2

W

Food and Description	Measure or Quantity	Calories
WAFFELOS, cereal (Ralston Purina)	1 cup	110
WAFFLE, frozen:		
(Aunt Jemima) jumbo	1 waffle	86
(Eggo):		
Apple cinnamon	1 waffle	150
Blueberry or strawberry	1 waffle	130
Home style	1 waffle	120
WALNUT, English or Persian		
(Diamond A)	1 cup	679
WALNUT FLAVORING, black		
(Durkee) imitation	1 tsp.	4
WATER CHESTNUT, canned:		
(Chun King) whole, drained	½ of 8½-oz. can	85
(La Choy) drained	¼ cup	16
WATERCRESS, trimmed	½ cup	3
WATERMELON:		
Wedge	4″ × 8″ wedge	111
Diced	½ cup	21
WELSH RAREBIT:		
Home recipe	1 cup	415
Frozen:		
(Green Giant)	5-oz. serving	219
(Stouffer's)	5-oz. serving	355
WENDY'S		
Bacon, breakfast	1 strip	55
Bacon cheeseburger on white bun	1 burger	460
Breakfast sandwich	1 sandwich	370
Buns:		
Wheat, multi-grain	1 bun	135
White	1 bun	160
Chicken sandwich on multi-grain bun	1 sandwich	320
Chili:		
Regular	8 oz.	260
Large	12 oz.	390
Condiments:		
Bacon	½ strip	30
Cheese, American	1 slice	70
Onion rings	.3-oz. piece	4
Pickle, dill	4 slices	1

Food and Description	Measure or Quantity	Calories
Relish	.3-oz. serving	14
Tomato	1 slice	2
Danish	1 piece	360
Drinks:		
Coffee	6 fl. oz.	2
Cola:		
Regular	12 fl. oz	110
Dietetic	12 fl. oz.	Tr.
Fruit flavored drink	12 fl. oz.	110
Hot chocolate	6 fl. oz.	100
Milk:		
Regular	8 fl. oz.	150
Chocolate	8 fl. oz.	210
Non-cola	12 fl. oz.	100
Orange juice	6 fl. oz.	80
Egg, scrambled	1 order	190
Frosty dairy dessert:		
Small	12 fl. oz.	400
Medium	16 fl. oz.	533
Large	20 fl. oz.	667
Hamburger:		
Double, on white bun	1 burger	560
Kids Meal	1 burger	220
Single:		
On wheat bun	1 burger	340
On white bun	1 burger	350
Omelet:		
Ham & cheese	1 omelet	250
Ham, cheese & mushroom	1 omelet	290
Mushroom, onion & green pepper	1 omelet	210
Potato:		
Baked, hot stuffed:		
Plain	1 potato	250
Broccoli & cheese	1 potato	500
Cheese	1 potato	590
Chicken à la King	1 potato	350
Sour cream & chives	1 potato	460
Stroganoff & sour cream	1 potato	490
French fries	regular order	280
Home fries	1 order	360
Salad Bar, Garden Spot:		
Alfalfa sprouts	2 oz.	20
Bacon bits	⅛ oz.	10
Blueberries, fresh	1 T.	8
Breadstick	1 piece	20
Broccoli	½ cup	14
Cantaloupe	1 piece (2 oz.)	4
Carrot	¼ cup	12
Cauliflower	½ cup	14

172

Food and Description	Measure or Quantity	Calories
Cheese:		
American, imitation	1 oz.	70
Cheddar, imitation	1 oz.	90
Cottage	½ cup	110
Mozzarella, imitation	1 oz.	90
Swiss, imitation	1 oz.	80
Chow mein noodles	¼ cup	60
Coleslaw	½ cup	90
Crouton	1 piece	2
Cucumber	¼ cup	4
Mushroom	¼ cup	6
Onions, red	1 T.	4
Orange, fresh	1 piece	5
Pasta salad	½ cup	134
Peas, green	½ cup	60
Peaches, in syrup	1 piece	8
Peppers:		
Banana or mild pepperoncini	1 T.	18
Bell	¼ cup	4
Jalapeño	1 T.	9
Pineapple chunks in juice	½ cup	80
Tomato	1 oz.	6
Turkey ham	¼ cup	46
Watermelon, fresh	1 piece (1 oz.)	1
Salad dressing:		
Regular:		
Blue cheese	1 T.	60
French, red	1 T.	70
Italian, golden	1 T.	45
Oil	1 T.	130
Ranch	1 T.	80
Thousand Island	1 T.	70
Dietetic:		
Bacon & tomato	1 T.	45
Cucumber, creamy	1 T.	50
Italian	1 T.	25
Thousand Island	1 T.	45
Wine vinegar	1 T.	2
Salad, Side, pick-up window	1 salad	110
Salad, taco	1 salad	390
Sausage	1 patty	200
Toast:		
Regular, with margarine	1 slice	125
French	1 slice	200
WESTERN DINNER, frozen:		
(Banquet) American Favorites	11-oz. dinner	513
(Morton) regular	11⅛-oz. dinner	347
(Swanson) *Hungry Man*	17½-oz. dinner	750
WHEATENA, cereal	¼ cup	112

Food and Description	Measure or Quantity	Calories
WHEAT FLAKES CEREAL		
(Featherweight)	1¼ cups	100
WHEAT GERM CEREAL		
(Kretschmer)	¼ cup	110
WHEAT GERM, RAW (Elam's)	1 T.	28
WHEAT HEARTS, cereal		
(General Mills)	1 oz.	110
WHEATIES, cereal	1 cup	110
WHEAT & OATMEAL CEREAL,		
hot (Elam's)	1 oz.	105
WHISKEY SOUR COCKTAIL		
(Mr. Boston)	3 fl. oz.	120
***WHISKEY SOUR MIX**		
(Bar-Tender's)	3½ fl. oz.	177
WHITE CASTLE:		
Bun only	.9-oz. bun	74
Cheese only	1 piece	31
Cheeseburger	1 sandwich	200
Chicken sandwich	1 sandwich	186
Fish sandwich	1 sandwich	155
French fries	1 order	301
Hamburger	1 sandwich	161
Onion chips	1 order	329
Onion rings	1 order	245
Sausage & egg sandwich	1 sandwich	322
Sausage sandwich	1 sandwich	196
WHITEFISH, LAKE:		
Baked, stuffed	4 oz.	244
Smoked	4 oz.	176
WIENER WRAP (Pillsbury)	1 piece	60
WILD BERRY DRINK,		
canned (Hi-C)	6 fl. oz.	88
WINCHELL'S DONUT HOUSE:		
Buttermilk, old fashioned	2-oz. piece	249
Cake, devil's food, iced	2-oz. piece	241
Cinnamon crumb	2-oz. piece	240
Iced, chocolate	2-oz. piece	227
Raised, glazed	1¾-oz. piece	212
WINE (See specific type, such as CHIANTI, SHERRY, etc.)		
WINE, COOKING (Regina):		
Burgundy or sauterne	¼ cup	2
Sherry	¼ cup	20
WINE COOLER (Bartles & Jaymes):		
Original white	6 oz.	92
Premium berry	6 oz.	92
Premium red	6 oz.	97

Y

Food and Description	Measure or Quantity	Calories
YEAST, BAKER'S (Fleischmann's):		
Dry, active	1 packet	20
Fresh & household, active	.6-oz. cake	15
YOGURT:		
Regular:		
Plain:		
(Dannon):		
Low-fat	8-oz. cont.	110
Non-fat	8-oz. cont.	140
(Friendship)	8-oz. container	170
(Johanna)	8-oz. container	150
Lite-Line (Borden)	8-oz. container	140
(Meadow Gold)	8-oz. container	160
(Whitney's)	6-oz. container	150
Yoplait	6-oz. container	130
Plain with honey, *Yoplait, Custard Style*	6-oz. container	160
Apple:		
(Dannon) Dutch *Fruit-on-the-bottom*	8-oz. container	240
Yoplait	6-oz. container	190
Apple-cinnamon, *Yoplait, Breakfast Yogurt*	6-oz. container	240
Apple & raisins (Whitney's)	6-oz. container	200
Apricot (Bison)	8-oz. container	262
Banana:		
(Dannon) *Fruit-on-the-bottom*	8-oz. container	240
LeShake (Kellogg's)	8-oz. container	170
Banana-Strawberry (Colombo)	8-oz. container	235
Berry (New Country) mixed	8-oz. container	210
Blueberry:		
(Bison):		
Regular	8-oz. container	262
Light	6-oz. container	162
(Breyer's)	8-oz. container	260
(Dannon) *Fresh Flavors*	8-oz. container	200
(Mountain High)	8-oz. container	220
(New Country) supreme	8-oz. container	210
(Riché)	6-oz. container	180

Food and Description	Measure or Quantity	Calories
(Sweet'N Low)	8-oz. container	150
(Whitney's)	6-oz. container	200
Yoplait	6-oz. container	190
Boysenberry:		
(Dannon)	8-oz. container	240
(Sweet'N Low)	8-oz. container	150
Cherry:		
(Breyer's) black	8-oz. container	270
(Dannon)	8-oz. container	240
(Friendship)	8-oz. container	230
(Riché)	6-oz. container	180
(Sweet 'n Low)	8-oz. container	150
Yoplait	6-oz. container	150
Cherry-vanilla (Colombo)	8-oz. container	250
Citrus, *Yoplait, Breakfast Yogurt*	6-oz. container	250
Coffee:		
(Colombo; Dannon)	8-oz. container	200
(Johanna)	8-oz. container	220
Exotic fruit (Dannon)	8-oz. container	240
Fruit crunch (New Country)	9-oz. container	210
Guava (Colombo)	8-oz. container	240
Hawaiian salad (New Country)	8-oz. container	210
Honey vanilla (Colombo)	8-oz. container	220
Lemon:		
(Dannon) *Fresh Flavors*	8-oz. container	200
(New Country) supreme	8-oz. container	210
(Sweet'N Low)	8-oz. container	150
(Whitney's)	6-oz. container	200
Yoplait:		
Regular	6-oz. container	190
Custard Style	6-oz. container	180
Mixed berries (Dannon):		
Extra Smooth	4.4-oz. container	130
Fruit-on-the-Bottom	8-oz. container	240
Orange, *Yoplait*	6-oz. container	190
Orange supreme (New Country)	8-oz. container	210
Orchard, *Yoplait,*		
Breakfast Yogurt	6-oz. container	240
Peach:		
(Breyer's)	8-oz. container	270
(Dannon)	8-oz. container	240
(Friendship)	8-oz. container	240
Lite-Line (Borden)	8-oz. container	230
(Meadow Gold) sundae style	8-oz. container	260
(New Country) 'n cream	8-oz. container	240
(Riché)	6-oz. container	180
(Sweet'N Low)	8-oz. container	150
(Whitney's)	6-oz. container	200
Peach melba (Colombo)	8-oz. container	230

Food and Description	Measure or Quantity	Calories
Piña colada:		
(Dannon)	8-oz. container	240
(Friendship)	8-oz. container	230
Pineapple:		
(Breyer's)	8-oz. container	270
(Light n' Lively)	8-oz. container	240
Raspberry:		
(Breyer's) red	8-oz. container	260
(Dannon):		
Extra Smooth	4.4-oz. container	130
Fresh Flavors	8-oz. container	200
(Light n' Lively) red	8-oz. container	230
(Riché)	6-oz. container	180
(Sweet'N Low)	8-oz container	150
Yoplait:		
Regular	6-oz. container	190
Custard Style	6-oz. container	180
Raspberry ripple (New Country)	8-oz. container	240
Strawberry:		
(Breyer's)	8-oz. container	270
(Dannon) *Fresh Flavors*	8-oz. container	200
(Friendship)	8-oz. container	230
(Light n' Lively)	8-oz. container	240
Lite-Line (Borden)	8-oz. container	240
(Meadow Gold)	8-oz. container	270
(Whitney's)	6-oz. container	200
Yoplait	6-oz. container	190
Strawberry-banana (Light n' Lively)	8-oz. container	260
Strawberry colada (Colombo)	8-oz. container	230
Tropical fruit (Sweet'N Low)	8-oz. container	150
Vanilla:		
(Breyer's)	8-oz. container	230
(Dannon):		
Fresh Flavors	8-oz. container	220
Hearty nuts & raisins	8-oz. container	270
(Friendship)	8-oz. container	210
(Lar Rogurt)	6-oz. container	160
(New Country) french ripple	8-oz container	240
(Whitney's)	6-oz. container	200
Yoplait, Custard Style	6-oz. container	180
Frozen, hard:		
Banana, *Danny-in-a-Cup*	8-oz. cup	210
Boysenberry, *Danny-On-A-Stick*, carob coated	2½-fl.-oz. bar	140
Boysenberry swirl (Bison)	¼ of 16-oz. container	116
Cherry vanilla (Bison)	¼ of 16-oz. container	116

177

Food and Description	Measure or Quantity	Calories
Chocolate:		
(Bison)	¼ of 16-oz. container	116
(Colombo) bar, chocolate coated	1 bar	145
(Dannon):		
Danny-in-a-Cup	8-fl.-oz. cup	190
Danny-On-A-Stick, chocolate coated	2½-fl.-oz. bar	130
Chocolate chip (Bison)	¼ of 16-oz. container	116
Chocolate chocolate chip (Colombo)	4-oz. serving	150
Mocha (Colombo) bar	1 bar	80
Piña colada:		
(Colombo)	4-oz. serving	110
(Dannon):		
(*Danny-in-a-Cup*	8-oz. cup	210
Danny-On-A-Stick	2½-fl.-oz. bar	65
Raspberry, red (Dannon):		
Danny-in-a-Cup	8-oz. container	210
Danny-On-A-Stick, chocolate coated	2½-fl.-oz. bar	130
Raspberry swirl (Bison)	¼ of 16-oz. container	116
Strawberry:		
(Bison)	¼ of 16-oz. container	116
(Colombo):		
Regular	4-oz. serving	110
Bar	1 bar	80
(Dannon):		
Danny-in-a-Cup	8 fl. oz.	210
Danny-Yo	3½ fl. oz.	110
Vanilla:		
(Bison)	¼ of 16-oz. container	116
(Colombo):		
Regular	4-oz. serving	110
Bar, chocolate coated	1 bar	145
(Dannon):		
Danny-in-a-Cup	8 fl. oz.	180
Danny-On-A-Stick	2½-fl.-oz. bar	65
Danny-Yo	3½-oz. serving	110
Frozen, soft (Colombo)	6-fl.-oz. serving	130
YOGURT DRINK (Dannon) *Dan'up*	8 oz.	190

Z

Food and Description	Measure or Quantity	Calories
ZINFANDEL WINE (Louis M. Martini) regular vintage	3 fl. oz.	57
ZITI, FROZEN:		
(Morton) Light	11-oz. dinner	280
(Weight Watchers)	11¼-oz. meal	290
ZWEIBACK (Gerber: Nabisco)	1 piece	30